Dear Al,
   Thanks for writing such a beautiful and compelling article. Its reach was amazing. I truly appreciate your genuine interest in Lindsay's story. Enjoy the book.
Love,
Judi

The View

from

Four Foot Two

D1596359

Judi Markowitz

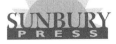
SUNBURY PRESS

Mechanicsburg, Pennsylvania   USA

Published by Sunbury Press, Inc.
50 West Main Street, Suite A
Mechanicsburg, Pennsylvania 17055

www.sunburypress.com

For information about special discounts for bulk purchases, please contact Sunbury Press Orders Dept. at (855) 338-8359 or orders@sunburypress.com.

To request one of our authors for speaking engagements or book signings, please contact Sunbury Press Publicity Dept. at publicity@sunburypress.com.

ISBN: 978-1-62006-288-3 (Trade Paperback)
ISBN: 978-1-62006-289-0 (Mobipocket)
ISBN: 978-1-62006-290-6 (ePub)

FIRST SUNBURY PRESS EDITION: December 2013

Product of the United States of America
0 1 1 2 3 5 8 13 21 34 55

Set in Bookman Old Style
Designed by Lawrence Knorr
Cover by Tammi Knorr
Edited by Jennifer Melendrez

Front cover image is of Lindsay Weiner at 3 years old.

Continue the Enlightenment!

Acknowledgments

I want to thank my friends and family for reading my manuscript at various stages of its development and providing valuable input. I am also deeply grateful for all the kind words of encouragement throughout this journey: Gayle and Ted Herkowitz, Alan and Cathy Foster, Shelley Jaffe, Barry, Barbara, and Jeff Kranitz, Benn Gilmore, Marty, Elise and Gideon Levinson, Mel and Sherry Foster, Mary Lynn Harrison, Suzi Wiener, Beth Gursky, Andrea Sachs, Beth Arimond, Paul Kavieff, Chris Mayo, and Jacque Hammons.

I also want to thank my family for their unconditional support. Thanks for listening, reading and rereading each chapter as it unfolded. I love all of you very much: Jeffrey, Lindsay, Chad, Eli, Todd and Chana Tova.

To my favorite cousin Mel Foster – Thank you for generously giving your time to edit and organize my book. Your insight and expertise is truly appreciated.

To Jeff Austin –Thank you for meeting me at Caribou Coffee, listening to my story about Lindsay and typing the first 30 pages. After that I was home free.

To Benn Gilmore – My gratitude runs deep. Thank you for your expert advice concerning the book. Above all, and most importantly, thank you for saving Lindsay's life.

To Andrea Sachs – Thank you for your guidance and introduction to the world of publishing.

To Paul Kavieff - Thanks for your inspiring words; you kept my spirits high and told me to persevere.

To Jennifer Melendrez – Thank you for your invaluable commentary and vision. Your direction is truly appreciated. Sunbury Press is fortunate to have such a talented editor.

To Lawrence and Tammi Knorr – Thank you for embracing this book. Your skill and integrity is above reproach. Thank you for answering my endless questions. "Continue the Enlightenment"

Dedication

For my family – You have enriched my life;
you are my world.

For Jeffrey, my wonderful husband, my best
friend and soul mate.

For Lindsay, Chad, Eli, Todd, Chana Tova
and our beautiful grand-daughters,
Shoshana Leiba, Tziporah Rochel and Shifra
Leah. You have given me more than words
can ever describe. I am truly grateful.

Introduction

There are 30 million people around the world with syndromes you have never heard of—Weaver, Soto's, Stickler, and Ehlers-Danlos Type III, to name just a few. And, there are 30 million mothers who, like me, were informed of the syndrome their baby was born with in words that sounded something like this:

> Your child is not normal. Blah, blah, blah. Your child will be different from all the other children. Blah, blah, blah. Those eyes you're staring into right now belong to someone who's damaged. It is not your fault. Or, maybe it is your fault. Blah, blah, blah. You have just delivered a functioning baby, but you have also delivered yourself a life sentence.

Some mothers, like me, whose children were born with Marshall-Smith Syndrome, also heard these words: "We have no record of a child with this syndrome living beyond the age of two."

Sometimes these words are delivered with compassion and sorrow. And sometimes they're delivered no differently than a diagnosis of heartburn.

My first child, Lindsay, was born with Marshall-Smith Syndrome in 1979. I can still hear the doctor's words when I shut my eyes at night. I did not completely understand them at the time. I do now. Denial has coalesced into reality with a brutal vengeance. It affected my life and the life of every person I have ever known and loved.

This year, I decided it was time to share a mother's story to celebrate the miracle of Lindsay and, hopefully, to remind every mother of a "normal" child never to take their miracles for granted.

Chapter One

"We think there's something wrong with Lindsay. We don't know what, but we're pretty sure something is wrong."

I was 27 years old and this was my first child. Natural childbirth was all the rage in 1979—every expectant mother I knew had read *Thank You, Dr. Lamaze* and attended Lamaze classes to learn the good doctor's breathing and delivery techniques. We felt somehow superior to our own mothers, who had relied on sedatives and anesthesia to get them through childbirth.

I was three weeks past my due date. At the time, however, there didn't seem to be much concern. I had undergone a pelvimetry exam (measurements of an x-rays image to determine shape and dimension of the pelvis) and the doctors assured me that everything was normal.

Looking back, I'm not sure that Lindsay wanted to arrive. She was a forceps delivery and immediately afterward there didn't seem to be much conversation in the delivery room. The APGAR test and the suctioning were performed and she was placed in my arms, tightly swaddled, with a small cap on her head. Silence. Lindsay weighed six pounds, nine ounces and she did not have a bit of baby fat. Once she did arrive, however, I'll never forget those huge eyes looking up at me as if to say, "I'm here and I'm not going anywhere." I believed I was staring into the most beautiful eyes I'd ever seen.

After a bit of bonding time, she was taken to the nursery and I was wheeled to a double room at Sinai

Hospital, the other bed occupied by a woman who had also just delivered. She, too, had used the Lamaze method.

In my case, all the techniques I'd learned flew out the window when labor began. The back pain was unbearable. Staying focused and breathing in a deep, rhythmic manner had no effect at all. I desperately wanted a Demerol, like the "unenlightened" women of my mother's generation, but even that didn't help. After 13 hours of labor, I was told that Lindsay should probably have been delivered C-section. I was torn apart from an episiotomy at the time. And I remembered thinking that the good doctor's book should probably be re-titled *Fuck You, Dr. Lamaze.*

"Lindsay has no body fat. She's very long. She has those wide eyes and an unusual face. However, not all babies come out looking perfect and she could wind up being the prom queen of her high school."

The words weren't making sense. The only birth defect I knew about back then was Down syndrome—of course, in 1979 everyone was less politically correct and I asked my doctor, "Is my baby a mongoloid?" Before he could answer, images flooded my mind—of trips I'd taken in 11th grade psychology class to a "mental institution" where "crazy" people were basically warehoused, confined to their wards, and written off by their families.

"Her eyes don't appear to have the shape of a Down syndrome baby," he said, "but we'll have to do a kariotype of her chromosomes to rule it out."

A woman experiences a wide range of emotions after giving birth. I think I covered the entire spectrum but, more often than not, I kept coming back to sadness. The moments when I should have been experiencing profound joy were filled with too many unknowns, and the trip from uncertainty to sadness was a short one.

I'm a very private person. I discussed the situation with only a few people who were very close to both me and my husband, Neil. After all, why would I discuss the possibility of there being something wrong with my beautiful, firstborn child when she could be a prom queen in 18 years? Optimism is my mainstay and this, too, kicked in with a vengeance. I couldn't wait to get out of that hospital and take my daughter to her new home where there would be a safe environment and no oppressive silence.

The woman who occupied the bed next to me rolled over after the doctor left the room and said, "I don't see anything wrong with your baby. She looks fine to me." I held onto those words during the next week while preparing myself mentally for Lindsay's first visit to the pediatrician.

Chapter Two

"Her chromosomes are perfectly normal. But we don't think she is."

We chose a pediatrician based on the recommendation of some close friends. They said the doctors in the practice they used were great, knowledgeable, informative, and caring. I should also point out that their children were all perfectly normal. A child like Lindsay has a way of recalibrating your judgment scale.

I was nervous before this first visit, and the moment I walked into the office, I felt that all eyes were on me. The medical assistant just happened to be a classmate of mine from high school and I had the odd feeling that my cover was blown. She obviously knew that something might be wrong with Lindsay. It bothered me. A lot. Still, I smiled and asked how she was, all the while thinking, "She read the chart. She knows there's something going on." Was I overly sensitive? Yes, but who wouldn't be, given the situation?

When the doctors came into the examination room they delivered the good news/bad news. Normal chromosomes/ abnormal baby. And then they did something that quite simply astounded me. They brought out various medical books and began leafing through the pages, studying photos of newborns with various syndromes and diseases. They were trying to find a match for Lindsay! It was the most absurd situation I had ever been in. Every once in a while, they paused over a photo, read the accompanying description, and moved on. They considered Pierre Robin Syndrome, floppy epiglottis, and stridor—the latter two dealing with noisy respirations. Lindsay definitely had loud breathing. In the end, however, we were sent home with no diagnosis and no reassuring words.

Along with natural childbirth, I had hoped to breastfeed my baby. The doctors strongly recommended against it since Lindsay was so thin—and it also appeared that she was not very interested, either. Every time I attempted to feed her it was almost comical. Lindsay would just stare at me with an expression that seemed to ask, "Huh?" Unfortunately, my breasts were engorged and they felt like rocks because Lindsay wasn't consuming enough. Finally, we resorted to bottle feeding so that Lindsay would receive the important vitamins and nutrients in the formula. She definitely needed to gain weight. So, we bought Playtex Nursers, the newest thing on the market back then for the "efficient" bottle feeding mother. It was official: as an "all-natural" mother, *I was a complete flop.*

Lindsay and I returned to the pediatrician's office the next week. The doctors commented on the slightness of her weight gain—and the medical books came out again. The show began. A repeat performance in absurdity. Finally, the pediatricians—whom I had naively assumed knew all the answers—shrugged and recommended that we see a geneticist at the University of Michigan who might be able to enlighten us. Their parting comment was not at all encouraging. "Don't worry, they'll find a syndrome for her."

We made an appointment with Dr. Roy Schmickel at Mott Children's Hospital in Ann Arbor. He was a very kind man and basically took down a lot of information regarding Lindsay's birth and her unusual appearance. Lindsay made snorting sounds at times when breathing in, and the doctor suggested she might have floppy epiglottis, a condition that can usually be corrected by medication. He said he wanted to keep an eye on Lindsay to make sure her breathing was not obstructed.

Being first-time parents, we were woefully inexperienced. I did not place Lindsay on her stomach for sleeping, as most other mothers did back then. There were many occasions when I placed her on her back and, as it turns out, this was most likely her saving grace for many months. I suppose I was ahead of the times with this positioning, but I did it only because it helped with her breathing issues. On her next visit, Dr. Schmickel said, "If she was my child, I would say that everything was fine."

Those words were Thanksgiving, Hanukkah, and World Peace all rolled into one. I'm not sure my mouth was capable of expanding wide enough to contain my smile. A thousand ton weight had just been lifted from my shoulders. I'm sure several tears escaped as well.

The doctor recommended that Lindsay have a full body scan to make sure everything was OK before we left the hospital. She had a very small, almost nonexistent chin and he wanted to be certain there were no obstructions to her breathing passages.

The elation Neil and I felt as we drove home that day turned out to be short-lived. A few days later, Dr. Schmickel's office called recommending that Lindsay be brought to the hospital for several days of observation. The x-ray had revealed that she had advanced bone age. I didn't have a clue what that was, but my mind leapt straight to an article I had read the week before in *The Detroit News*. There was a picture of a young lady, 20 years old, who looked as though she was 80. She suffered from a condition known as Progeria—rapid aging. People afflicted with this condition rarely live past 20 and, in fact, many die well before that. There is no known cure. Was this to be the fate of my firstborn child?

I packed two days' worth of clothing plus Lindsay's favorite swing and drove to Ann Arbor. Only my immediate family knew why we were going. Friends were told we were leaving for a short family trip because, once again, my optimism steeled itself to do battle with reality.

While filling out the admission forms, there, in bold letters, were the words "Marshall-Smith Syndrome" in the space labeled "diagnosis." These words would haunt and mystify me from that time on. What the hell was Marshall-Smith Syndrome? Why weren't Neil and I told about this diagnosis? What, in God's name, did it mean? The lofty vision I had of the medical community once again came crashing down to earth.

When Lindsay was finally situated in the nursery, Dr. Schmickel arrived. I'm not sure we made it much past, "Hello," before I asked, "OK, what is Marshall-Smith Syndrome?"

His response was brief and businesslike. He stated that Lindsay wasn't a classic case and that the radiologist was the one who discovered the condition. Children with Marshall-Smith have a bone age that is older than their chronological age. Lindsay's bone age at two months was that of a three to five year old, he explained. What did this mean? Nobody knew. The trip to Ann Arbor, he assured me, was simply to observe Lindsay, her breathing, her feeding habits, and to take a sample of her skin to freeze so that in years to come they might learn something.

I couldn't help wondering what they expected to learn, however, if there was nothing really wrong to begin with.

"Marshall-Smith Syndrome consists of multiple congenital anomalies."

No procedures were performed during the first day. The next morning, however, a geneticist, followed by a group of new residents, came to examine Lindsay. Boy, did this guy need a lesson in bedside manner. "Marshall-Smith Syndrome features advanced bone age as well as severe retardation," he explained. They looked. They gawked. They felt just as uncomfortable as I did, but they were much too young to know the pain of a first-time mother. Their mentor was the poster child for abominable bedside manner, lacking both sensitivity and tact. He had absolutely no idea how deeply those two words had stabbed me. Severe retardation. Now I knew something else about a syndrome they knew "nothing" about. Things were going from bad to worse.

After they left the room, I called a friend in medical school as well as my brother-in-law, who is an optometrist. Personal computers were virtually nonexistent then, as was easy access to the Internet. Computers could only be reserved through a large library by someone with proper credentials. Eventually, as a result of those calls, we received a hard copy of several medical articles. One had sparse information and photos as well. The other article was written in German with lengthy details concerning Marshall-Smith Syndrome. I had taken two years of German in high school and I translated every word in that article with the aid of my old English-German dictionary. Those words became my mantra for the next few months. "Marshall-Smith Syndrome consists of multiple congenital anomalies." I looked up "anomalies" in Webster's Dictionary and broke out in a sweat. Basically, it meant my daughter had birth defects that were insurmountable.

I read the translation of that article over and over again, as if to torture myself. It was inconceivable to me that my daughter was like the two children featured as examples. It seemed as if they purposely intended to take the worst possible photos of these kids and put them in the article merely for shock value. However, the most terrifying part of the article was that these two children died at an early age. In fact, the author hypothesized that no child with this syndrome would live past 20 months.

Another article from January, 1971, stated:

Two cases of accelerated osseous maturation and relative failure to thrive are reported as a newly recognized entity, the eventual elucidation of which may yield knowledge pertinent to the regulation of skeletal maturation. Case 1. Patient D.C. was born to 24-year-old Caucasian parents after an uneventful pregnancy. He weighed 3,300 gm and was 50 cm long. He was noted to have an unusual facies with bulging eyes, coarse eyebrows, low nasal bridge, and an umbilical hernia. His immediate course was characterized by noisy respirations, copious nasal secretions, and difficulty in breathing. His development was severely delayed; and by 20 months he could not walk and had only a two word vocabulary. He had frequent upper respiratory infections for which no cause was determined. He suddenly died at 20 months of age. Postmortem examination revealed hemorrhagic pneumonia with no bacterial growth by culture. His brain revealed broad convolutions in the occipitoparietal area, suggestive of pachygyria with no microscopic abnormalities. The morphology and history of the other organs were considered to be normal.

After reading about D.C. I was paralyzed, but I had to read on.

Case 2. Patient M.F. had pneumonia at 7 months of age and responded slowly to antibiotic therapy. His development has been retarded; at 6 months he could not support his head and was unable to roll over, and at 10 months he could not sit, creep, or use a single word. At 10 months there was further evidence of skeletal abnormality; he had developed a flexion contracture of the distal phalanx on his fifth left finger and a left lumbodorsal scoliosis.

This was simply too profound to comprehend. All I could think was that a death sentence had just been placed on Lindsay in the form of Marshall-Smith Syndrome. She needed help. I needed help. There had to be a way to avoid her becoming Case 3.

After reading the German articles, I called Dr. Schmickel and confronted him with the fact that he had withheld all of this information from us. Did he really think we lived in a bubble? His warmth and sensitivity flowed forward, however, and he stated once again that Lindsay was not a classic case. It was possible that Lindsay did not have all of the complications and malformations that were evident in the other children, he told us. I heard him. But I also heard that it was possible she *did* have all the problems evident in Case 1 and Case 2.

Shortly after this conversation I received a letter from Dr. Schmickel. His compassion was heartfelt. He stated:

I believe that these past few months have been very difficult for you. However, I also believe that you have achieved a deep and thorough understanding of the situation you face. Although you are realistic, you are also hopeful. I believe this is appropriate. The hardest lesson to learn is how to live with the unknown and still not accept it as an absolute. The highest art of living is to enjoy the present when the future is uncertain.

His message was appreciated.

Neil and I kept the words "Marshall-Smith Syndrome" to ourselves. Grandparents were not apprised of the major details and neither were friends. We did, however, tell our siblings. Everyone who came to see Lindsay sensed that *something* wasn't right.

No one actually said anything—after all, how could a close friend call up and say, "Yeah, hey, just wondering … is there something wrong with your child?" They were afraid and so were we. My silence was a helpful tool, because if I never told anyone that Lindsay had a syndrome, then maybe that would manifest itself into the truth.

Chapter Three

"I want it to go away, God. That's not too much to ask, is it?"

I can remember walking down the halls of Oak Park High School as a student, looking up at the ceiling, and thanking God for my wonderful life. I would pray to do well on tests, and God would answer my prayers.

Now, the God that I'd believed in, who was merciful and wonderful—my lifelong advocate—was playing a horrible trick on me. Did I do something horribly wrong, I wondered? Did Neil? Was I more sinful than most kids? I began to analyze every aspect of my life. I began to pray to God for Lindsay. I wanted everything to change and I wanted Marshall-Smith Syndrome to go away. After all, I was a pretty decent person—a good child to my parents with only minor infractions along the way, a good student, and a good wife. I couldn't figure out why this was happening.

Since I told no one about Lindsay's diagnosis, I had no one to confide in, except God. I couldn't believe He was responsible for all the ills in the world and I kept asking why this had to happen to Lindsay. Marshall-Smith Syndrome affected one child in a million. So why Lindsay? Since I grew up in an era when mostly boys went to Hebrew school, I can truly say that I didn't have enough knowledge about my own religion to feel satisfied with God's treatment of my daughter. The more I pondered the situation, the more disillusioned I became with this God I had held in such high esteem. Still, I continued to pray.

As I looked down at little Lindsay, I couldn't imagine that same ill fate befalling her as befell those poor children in the German literature. I started to wonder if maybe something else could help me.

I began to contemplate if, maybe, Jesus could heal my baby. I was grasping at anything—after all, Jesus was Jewish, right? The main thing I knew about the New Testament was that Jesus performed miracles, and now was certainly the time for a huge one. His name was promptly entered into my prayers as well, and I begged Jesus to save Lindsay. I needed strength and I needed it right away.

Jews for Jesus started knocking on my door. So did Jehovah's Witnesses, and I answered. Ironically, they were in the neighborhood proselytizing at the time I was at my absolute lowest. I might have been grasping at straws by speaking to them, but at least it appeared that I had new forces to help me and to help Lindsay. After a year, however, I grew disillusioned with these groups and returned to the familiarity of Judaism.

In 1981, Rabbi Harold S. Kushner wrote a book entitled, *When Bad Things Happen to Good People*. It was an overnight success. Those looking for answers, guidance, and general information on dealing with life's difficult situations found this book helpful. Rabbi Kushner didn't proclaim to know the *why*s and *wherefore*s of life's most perplexing situations; however, he did craft a philosophy that helped him during his most trying times.

His son, Aaron, was born with a rare condition known as Progeria—a rare genetic condition that produces rapid aging in children. The rabbi wrote:

> I knew that one day I would write this book. I would write it out of my own need to put into words some of the most important things I have come to believe and know. And I would write it to help other people who might one day find themselves in a similar predicament. I would write for all those

people who wanted to go on believing, but whose anger at God made it hard for them to hold onto their faith and be comforted by religion. And I would write it for all those people whose love for God and devotion to Him led them to blame themselves for their suffering and persuade themselves that they deserved it.

I certainly could relate to these thoughts since I had been whirling with conflicted views of life, God, and the uncertainty of the future. Like Lindsay, Aaron was dealt an unfortunate hand. Progeria was the very thing that I'd thought Lindsay suffered from when I was told about her advanced bone age. Progeria caused rapid aging of the organs which, in turn, expressed itself in an appearance of old age, short stature, loss of hair, and, ultimately, early death. Like me, the Kushner's had to sort out the unsortable and try to make sense of the senseless.

Since Harold Kushner was taught in the traditional Jewish manner, the assertions he made in his book were truly unconventional. Having gone through a life-altering ordeal, he questioned the will of God. Rabbi Kushner could no longer accept the teachings of traditional Judaism, accepting that God dictated every good and bad thing that happened in our lives. In order to persevere he needed to create a new perspective that made sense and felt right— even if it did not correspond with the traditional path he had followed for so many years.

Rabbi Kushner stated:

I believe in God. But I do not believe the same things about Him that I did years ago, when I was a theological student. I recognize His limitations. He is limited by what He can do, by laws of nature, and by evolution of human nature and human moral freedom. I no longer hold God responsible for illnesses, accidents, and natural disasters, because I realize that I gain little and I lose so much when I blame God for those things.

This philosophy helped the rabbi through a dark period in his life and gave him a new outlook in order to move forward.

If Rabbi Kushner's perspective has helped many people then it is a positive act in a world that's quite complicated. But, after soul searching for many years, I simply could not abandon the notion of a God who *is* in total control of this universe, whether we like it or not. Now, 30 years later, I have finally surrendered to the belief that I may not know God's purpose, but I do know that God is with me and my family.

When placed in difficult situations, each of us has to make decisions. After Lindsay's birth I began to take inventory of my life—not only those situations that pertained to me, but those of friends, acquaintances, and colleagues as well. It became quite clear that no one goes through this life unscathed. We all have our battles; some are minor and others are fought on unforgiving terrain. We also have choices, however—choices in the manner in which we conduct ourselves during these battles. For me, it basically boiled down to just two: I could allow myself to be consumed with grief, or I could face the hard, cold facts and move forward. There was no gray area here. I chose to enjoy life with Lindsay, whatever that might hold.

I truly believe that due to all of my prayers—and anyone else who prayed for Lindsay—that I *was* given a miracle. It just took a while to recognize this. There were only 18 cases of MSS reported in the world's medical literature by 1982, when Lindsay turned five—and she was alive. By beating these statistics, God had granted her the opportunity to be something special and *that* was the miracle.

"I couldn't take Lindsay back to the page-flipping pediatricians."

My sister's friend recommended a new pediatrician. I was optimistic about this appointment, especially now that I had more information about Lindsay's condition. After all, he might be able to offer some encouraging advice.

While filling out the usual forms in the waiting room and writing those awful words, Marshall-Smith Syndrome, however, I started to get nervous. I tried to ignore it. I always tried to keep such feelings in check until I was alone.

Upon entering the examination room, there were smiles all around. I shared Lindsay's background information with the doctor realizing, as I spoke, he knew nothing about this condition. Realizing, too, that most doctors were probably in the same situation. I had put doctors on a pedestal. After all, they went to college for eight years— shouldn't they know everything? Nonetheless, it took me a while to comprehend that they were just like me: they were people on a learning curve, no more, no less.

The doctor excused himself after a cursory exam and left the room. When he returned, there was that damn book again. This time, however, it had a different title: *Human Malformations*. He had to look up the condition and, low and behold, there was one more horrid picture of a child born with Marshall-Smith Syndrome. (As if I needed to see another picture and read more information in this collection of oddities.) After reading a few paragraphs, he stated: "*If* she makes it, we can talk about possible, beneficial therapies."

And that was the end of pediatrician number two.

Chapter Four

"Neil began to withdraw both physically and emotionally."

They say when an irresistible force meets an immovable object, something has to give. Lindsay was the force; my marriage (I thought) was the immovable object. Neil and I were just 22 years old when we married. I was already teaching in a middle school and Neil was still in college. In retrospect, our marriage was very much like an amusement park ride—the jolting up and down motion of a rollercoaster. When things were good, we would sail smoothly over those tracks. However, the sharp turns and rapid speed eventually caused our marriage to derail.

Outwardly, it seemed like we were a happy couple and well suited for one another. It was a facade, however, and one that went on way too long. We had dated on and off for many years and then we married, well, because it was the thing to do. Early on, I grew unhappy with our marriage but still tried to focus on the positives. And I hoped for change. After five years of marriage, change came in the form of a baby girl named Lindsay.

Neil definitely loved Lindsay and was her advocate right from the start. He called doctors, made inquiries, and was hungry for details. When I became depressed with all of the devastating information concerning Marshall-Smith Syndrome, Neil maintained a positive attitude. Conversely, I would be there to cheer him up when he became overwhelmed. But when there were no answers and door after door was slammed shut, Neil began to withdraw both physically and emotionally.

Business trips often took him out of town for weeks on end. I think that the only reason our marriage endured as long as it did was due to the fact that Neil traveled so much. Phone conversations were pleasant and compensated for the many arguments we had at home. It was as if there was an alternate universe when he left on those business trips. On the phone, we could act with civility and pretend that all of our problems would somehow remedy themselves. We were living a lie. Neil and I simply didn't get along because we were on different wavelengths.

It was the 1970s, the Age of Aquarius and Women's Liberation, and yet I felt trapped in old traditions. Divorce danced through my mind, but I held this forbidden idea at bay. My dad told me many times that "our back door is always open to you." That had been his signal phrase to me when I was living at home. I would come in late from a date and always enter the house through the back door so as not to wake my parents. (But, as loving parents, they nevertheless remained awake until their daughter arrived home safely.) My dad sensed that the glory days were not shining down on his daughter and son-in-law. All was not kosher. His repetition of this signal phrase let me know I had a safe haven. And yet, in spite of this, I felt as though my feet were stuck in cement.

As I reflect back on this period in our marriage, my situation reminds me of Tim O'Brien, the main character in the novel, *The Things They Carried*, by Tim O'Brien. Tim put himself into the novel to show his pain and suffering during the Vietnam War. As a character, he was able to change the facts and thus manipulate the stories. It would be up to the reader to discern the truth.

In one of the chapters entitled, "On the Rainy River," Tim worked in a meat packing plant the summer of his graduation from college. He believed he wouldn't be drafted since he was about to enter graduate school. One day, however, he came home from work to find that his draft notice had arrived. Tim, extremely upset, packed a bag and headed north.

He lived in Minnesota, and the proximity to Canada was reassuring. After several hours, Tim came across the Tip Top Lodge and its owner, Elroy Berdahl. Tim asked about employment. He worked diligently and helped Elroy to close down the resort for the harsh winter season. At the end of the first week, Elroy and Tim went fishing on the Rainy River and Elroy navigated their boat within twenty yards of the Canadian coast. Elroy was affording Tim an opportunity to swim to the Canadian shore. At that point, however, Tim realized that Canada had become a "pitiful fantasy."

Tim said:

What embarrasses me much more, and always will, is the paralysis that took my heart. A moral freeze: I couldn't decide, I couldn't act ... All those eyes on me—the town, the whole universe—and I couldn't risk the embarrassment. It was as if there were an audience to my life ... I couldn't endure the mockery or the disgrace. I was a coward.

This was my own personal dilemma as well. I liked the idea of being an independent woman, making my own decisions; however, I couldn't pull the trigger on the most important issue in my life. I resolved to stay in a bad marriage because I did not want people to talk about me, just as Tim did not want his town to think that he was afraid of becoming a soldier. I, too, was a coward.

So, Neil and I had three more children together. And as each child was born, responsibilities mounted. Since Neil was gone so often I was the one to orchestrate everyone's routine. For doctor appointments, shopping, cooking, play dates, physical therapy, carpools, soccer, baseball, and basketball practice, I was in charge. And when Neil's travels brought him home, he never stayed long enough to dig his feet in and help with the routine. His friends and activities took him away and I simply continued with the job of nurturing our four children.

As a matter of fact, some business trips were extended because of a detour to Florida to visit a good buddy or a decision (not mine) to go to the Indy Five Hundred. Neil was also sighted at a convention in Las Vegas tanning himself by the pool, well before his business venture began. I do remember that when he arrived home from that trip he continued tanning on our deck while I took care of our children with the help of my parents. I could actually see the steam coming out of my father's ears. Many of these trips were "joy rides" while I was home embarking on the most important job in life. Sometimes I wondered if I had *five* children, not four.

We argued all the time. Neighbors could hear us when the windows were open. I was mortified, yet I couldn't back off. I just didn't understand why this man, my husband, could not reach down deep enough to help out with the children. He enjoyed the fun aspects of a large family—playing ball with the boys, going for bike rides and watching their games—but when it came to the tedious stuff like changing diapers or picking the kids up from school, he rarely had time. And those middle-of-the-night feedings for the babies were definitely out of the question. I was alone.

After visits to an array of marriage counselors, Neil and I remained polar opposites regarding family life. I needed a partner and a father for the children who could demonstrate his love instead of just mouthing it. What good is saying "I love you" if there's nothing to back it up? One therapist suggested that "tiny, baby steps" needed to be taken on Neil's behalf. I was told, "Give him space to adjust." Another said to "hire a driver to help with all the kids' activities." And yet another one stated that I should begin each request for help with the phrase, "I would appreciate it if _____." I was outraged with all three methods. After all, I didn't take baby steps to motherhood; it was a full, fathomless plunge. Why was Neil so different?

After nearly 20 years, we finally ended our marriage. I was the custodial parent and Neil promised to be with the kids more since it would now be on his terms. In our divorce agreement he was to spend every other weekend with all of the children at his apartment. As time went on, however, those weekend visits came to a screeching halt.

Though it sounds cliché, the best part of our marriage was the birth of our four children. However, the statistics were against us from the start. Things had been rocky even before Lindsay was born. The research in 1979 indicated that a couple with a disabled child had a 50% chance of making their marriage work. Today those odds apply to all marriages. In fact, according to one current study, the divorce rate for couples with a disabled child is now as high as 85-90%. Those statistics can be daunting to even the best of marriages.

An interesting comment from a parent in Dr. Laura Marshak's book, *Married with Special-Needs Children*, states:

> The advice I give to couples who sail into a storm and are fighting is: 'Don't hack at your boat in a storm. If you are in the middle of a crisis, don't take the very support you have and start whacking at it, because that is dumb. You should love, nurture, and care for the other person or you are not going to make it through the storm.'

Neil and I did not survive the onslaught. Our boat gradually sank.

Chapter Five

"I was determined to make each day beautiful for Lindsay and, in doing so, I was able to enjoy things."

Most mothers in the 70s and 80s put their careers on hold for a while to raise their children. We were ladies who lunched with our friends and children. Watching all those healthy kids reach their milestones was a killer for me. Yet, I persevered and went to every single event. I happily reciprocated and had all of my friends and their babies over to my house as well. The children were the epitome of health, and I marveled at this gift and wondered why Lindsay had been denied.

I once confided in my sister, telling her how difficult it was and she said, "Just don't do it anymore. Remove yourself from the loop." I couldn't. I had to live life to the fullest and I needed Lindsay to be immersed in it as well. Certainly, it would be easy to simply hide and wallow in my sorrow. The difficult part was moving forward, but I kept pushing in that direction no matter what. A quote from Helen Keller kept popping into my head: "Self-pity is our worst enemy and if we yield to it, we can never do anything good in the world."

So I proceeded with life as if Lindsay wasn't disabled. Don't think I was in denial; in order to enjoy my baby and maintain an even perspective I had no other choice except optimism. Believe me, I was aware—every single moment— of Lindsay's tenuous grasp on life. Most of the time I could push my feelings down so deep that it made it easier for me to proceed each day. Faced with the possibility of her death, as stated in the MSS literature, I refused to let those statistics occupy my mind because they would immobilize me and put me in a place of utter abandonment.

I was determined to make each day beautiful for Lindsay. In doing so, I was able to continue with my daily routines and enjoy life as much as possible. Of course, there would always be times when the utter unfairness of Lindsay's condition would come rushing through me and I couldn't stall the flow of despair. These moments were unpredictable and felt like a sledgehammer when they hit. I could be enjoying a day at the park, pushing Lindsay on a swing, then look across at another child and think, "My daughter should be able to do all of the things that child does. It's not fair." I was once told that having a child with disabilities and working through your feelings about it was similar to facing the death of a loved one. There are steps one must go through—grief, denial, anger, bargaining, and acceptance—in order to come to terms with the situation. However, no matter how far you push down your feelings or work through them in a healthy manner, these emotions never really go away.

There are always intervals of dramatic loss and sadness that surface without warning. Life milestones such as close friendships, dating, driving a car, college education, and marriage are all things that are beyond Lindsay's purview. Even when I attend an important social event for one of my friends or relatives and am enjoying the moment, I might reflect on her loss and the flood gates need to be reinforced. It's not exactly the right moment to pity myself or Lindsay and, of course, I have to pull it together before I'm detected. I can't allow such moments to linger too long because they are simply too sad. I need to remind myself constantly to focus on all of the good. I need to recognize that Lindsay is with her family, enjoying all these important occasions with people who love her very much. Lindsay was my daughter, my firstborn; she became Todd, Chad, and Eli's big sister; and it was my maternal obligation to make damn sure that her life was as full as possible. So I determined early on that she was to participate in all activities, no matter how difficult the situation.

There was never a time when Lindsay would stay home because one of the boys had a concert or a ballgame, or because we were going to the movies. Lindsay was always included since that's how life is: families do things *together*. Even though someone has a disability it doesn't mean they should be excluded. I must admit it wasn't always easy. Lindsay had to learn appropriate social behavior, and many times she had her own ideas of what was acceptable. We could be in line at a grocery store and she might start yelling. I would have to talk to her and tell her to calm down. This began a pattern where Lindsay would learn through doing. The more she participated in activities, the better she became at navigating social situations. Ninety percent of the time Lindsay is quite adept at having a feel for the people around her and the situation she finds herself in. She can detect if people are comfortable with her and, if not, she will become extremely shy. I might ask her to wave hello or ask her a question, but she won't respond because she truly picks up on people's feelings.

One issue in particular that has always been unnerving is when people stare at her. When my boys were younger and we were all out together, they would become very angry if they caught someone staring at Lindsay. I struggled with these feelings as well, but I quickly learned that people are uncomfortable with someone who is different. They don't know how to react and so they simply stare, trying to make sense of things. I try to turn such situations around. I might say hello or introduce Lindsay to those who are gawking and sometimes that might break the ice. Children are the worst offenders. After all, they're uneducated in the art of subtlety. Children will instinctively turn around or gaze at Lindsay for many an uncomfortable moment, until their parents discover the indiscretion and try to distract their attention. I have overheard many parents try to explain to their children that "some people are born with problems" or "that girl is one of God's children and she should be treated just like anyone else." I prefer the second explanation.

One of the most troubling of such occasions occurred during Halloween when Lindsay was ten years old. All of the kids were in costume and we were going from house to house trick-or-treating. The streets were teeming with children dressed in their finest costumes and it appeared that there was nothing but goodwill in the air—that is until a child who was walking past Lindsay said to her, "Great mask." Lindsay wasn't wearing one!

It took me a long time to reconcile my outrage at the ignorance of people, at their uncomfortable stares and rude comments. This didn't happen overnight. These situations unnerved me and I know they did the same to Todd, Chad, and Eli. After all, she was their sister and they were not going to tolerate disrespectful behavior. However, there were times when common sense flew out the window and the boys simply wanted to clobber anyone who looked at their sister the wrong way. I had to hold them back from staring someone down or saying something inappropriate. I reiterated to them that they needed to educate people with their actions, not hit them with their fists.

Ultimately, their actions have been filled with love and acceptance toward their sister. They have carved out an incredible life with Lindsay and have taught their friends to interact with her and talk to her like any other person. Brett, one of Eli's friends, will even come over from time-to-time and wait for Lindsay's bus to arrive so he can carry her into the house and simply hang out with her. This kind of love doesn't just happen; it is learned. I'm sure there were many times when the boys, like me, had to deal with accepting the fact that this happened to Lindsay; that she does have differences and that things are not always easy if she decides to have a meltdown. But, they understand that this is Lindsay's way of expressing herself, because she doesn't have language skills. They have the ability to take a step back and deal with the situation. And due to their involvement with her, Lindsay attended twelve straight years of basketball games at Berkley High School and was a loyal fan! She loved being part of the excitement! Her brothers would always come into the stands to give her a kiss in front of all their teammates. Every baseball, basketball, football, and soccer game, every choir performance and track meet, Lindsay was there for her brothers; and her brothers were proud of her.

Our family also travels quite a bit and people frequently ask, "Is Lindsay going?" By now, most have stopped asking that ridiculous question because of the obvious answer, "Yes, Lindsay is going. She is part of our family." She has traveled more places than most able-bodied people and does so skillfully. Lindsay enjoys the action: car rides, boat rides, and plane rides. She has more patience than most people I know, especially when waiting in line. Granted, it's not always easy, but Todd, Chad, and Eli take turns and they carry their sister down the aisle into her seat on the airplane and to any places that are not handicap accessible. As a matter of fact, Todd carried Lindsay to the Seven Sacred Pools in Maui because the road was filled with stones and it was impossible to push her wheelchair. She was also carried through some of the smaller tunnels under the Western Wall in Jerusalem by Chad due to the fact that her chair just wouldn't fit in such a confined area. Eli had the honor of dancing with Lindsay at Todd's wedding. He picked her up and whirled her around the floor so that she could enjoy herself. Her laughter was penetrating. The list is quite long, but Lindsay doesn't miss a beat. If there is an obstacle somewhere, it is usually overcome.

Together, our family has made it possible for Lindsay to live an action-packed life. I'm always cognizant of the fact that friends don't come knocking on the door for Lindsay, so I had to ensure that she was engaged in activities. Lindsay has enjoyed ice skating lessons with her aluminum walker to assist with balance, and she attended Horseback Riding for Handicappers (until her hips started becoming problematic). She has also participated in a bowling league at school. Adaptive equipment made it possible to place a bowling ball on a ramp so that Lindsay could push the ball, sending it down the lane. I'm an over-the-top energetic person and I have instilled this, too, in

Lindsay. In fact, she will take my hand when we're at home and walk me straight to the car to let me know she wants to go away. She has become a shopaholic and we have a great time! There's nothing more enjoyable than buying new clothes and watching Lindsay select the color and style. I simply hold up each item and she will put her hand on the one she likes best. Lindsay's quite adept at this and it's heartwarming. She's truly my buddy!

To carve out special time with the boys, I took advantage of volunteering at school, being a room parent, and going on field trips with their classes. Lunch dates were set and each child was picked up from school for a special treat. This was done on a regular basis. The boys needed my time as well, and I was happy to be there. These times worked out nicely since Lindsay was at school and no special arrangements had to be made for a caregiver. She attended a different school than the boys. When they had special days off of school, such as conferences or teacher professional development days, we would go to the movies. I tried to make time for each of them. However, with four children, individual time is hard to come by, and I knew I had to maximize my involvement in all of their activities. I consider myself lucky to have been immersed in their lives. I noticed there were so many mothers who were working and couldn't volunteer or find the time to even attend parent/teacher conferences. As for me, I couldn't imagine not being involved at every level.

"The Lindsay factor: I can no longer handle abusive parents or abusive parkers."

We have all heard the mantra, "Practically anyone can have a child, but not everyone is cut out to be a parent." No truer words were ever spoken. I have been in quite a few situations where I've observed parents smacking their children in public. I'm not talking about a little swat to straighten out a child's behavior. Oh no, I'm talking about out and out abusive behavior. I realize that people have to be cautious about approaching others and discussing issues like this with total strangers. However, every now and again I have found myself unable to resist.

The first time, I was appalled when I witnessed an adult (presumably the parent) smacking a small child in the back seat of a car that was parked close to mine. I was in the lot of a strip mall near my house. The sounds coming from that car were heartbreaking. I couldn't help but approach the car, and when I asked what he was doing I found myself staring into the eyes of a crazy man. I commented that his discipline was out of control and that he should leave the child alone. First he stared me down and then he began to get out of his car. When I observed him putting the little girl on the seat and reaching for the door, it was my cue to exit the scene quickly. I ran into the first store that I could and hid inside a fitting room, waiting for what seemed an eternity. A salesperson came by to see if I needed assistance with clothing, and I described the man who was tailing me. She became my lookout. He combed the store and when he didn't spot me, he walked out. It didn't matter to him that he left that little girl alone and unsupervised in the car. I was very lucky, to say the least, that we never met up again. I realize that I am overly sensitive about anybody hurting a child, but it's reprehensible that anyone would take their healthy child for granted. It's impossible for me to witness such behavior and stay silent.

A second incident occurred in a parking lot as well. I was getting Lindsay's wheelchair out of my car when I noticed a woman holding a baby in one arm and dragging another child with her other hand. When I say dragging I am not exaggerating. The little girl could not have been more than two years old and her knees were being torn apart by her "loving" mom. Now, we all know that small children can be quite a handful; however, this does not give anyone the right to harm them. This mother continued to drag her child to the car and then she proceeded to place her baby in the car seat. While doing so, she let go of her daughter. As it happened, the little girl started to move away from the car and then was pulled back by her ponytail. The woman noticed me looking at her. Other shoppers noticed as well.

No one said a word—until I opened up my mouth, that is. I looked straight at her as I was helping Lindsay into her wheelchair and I commented that she was abusing her daughter. She got into her car and drove over to me as I was walking with Lindsay across the parking lot. She rolled down her window and began to tell me a sob story. It was a tale of a little girl who behaved badly in the store for thirty minutes and would not listen to her mother. The "dragging" was necessary to ensure her well-being. She really seemed to believe this story but I wasn't buying it. I expressed concern over her abusive conduct once again, and told her that she should be grateful to have healthy children and to treat them with love and understanding. She said that she thanked God each night for her children. I couldn't take the bullshit anymore so I proceeded on my way.

Handicapped parking is yet another subject that brings out the crusader in me. When Lindsay was still quite small, I thought it might be a good idea to obtain a handicapped sticker for my car. After all, she was not walking at the time when most youngsters took off with wings on their feet, so I figured that accessibility was necessary, especially in inclement weather. I asked one of Lindsay's doctors for a prescription and took it to the Secretary of State. The process was easy—one simply presents the necessary documentation and pays a minimal fee. The date on the sticker really freaked me out, though. It was valid for five years. It was strange to see that number hanging in front of me every time I entered the car.

Once I received the sticker, however, life was a bit easier since navigating to a desirable spot in a parking lot was now a no-brainer.

My boys have commented at various times that having a handicapped sticker is the only perk for individuals with disabilities. However, I discovered, much to my dismay, that handicapped parking is not always accessible but not because the spaces are taken by people with legitimate parking stickers. Instead, there are many people who seem to believe that the sign with "Handicapped Parking " is meant for them, even if they don't have a sticker.

Some actually feel justified in taking a parking space away from a person who is physically impaired. I have circled around many lots in search of a legitimate space only to find someone sitting in their car without the necessary sticker. I like to think that I need to give these people the benefit of the doubt. Sometimes I even think that they might be driving the "other" family car—the one that doesn't have the sticker. (Although whenever that has happened to me, I usually decline to park illegally.) The people who feel they have the right to park without the handicapped sticker, however, are usually made from a very different mold. Not only do they feel it's all right to occupy these spaces for their convenience, most also do not care about the individual they are inconveniencing. A perfectly healthy driver can be sitting in a handicapped spot waiting for their partner and, when challenged, offer the most insulting responses.

I have approached many drivers with this question: "Excuse me, do you realize that you are in a handicapped parking spot and you do not have a sticker?" Many of the responses are similar in nature. "I'm just waiting for my wife. She's only running in for a moment and there weren't any spaces available." Or, "I'm waiting here because it's the closest spot available and I'll only be a minute."

With each reoccurring incident throughout the years I have felt insulted, hurt, dismayed, amazed, and simply disgusted by individuals who feel it is their God given right to park wherever they please. I think it's unfortunate that there aren't parking spaces reserved for these VIPs—Very Important Pricks. If such a category existed, there would be a lot of people deserving of this sticker!

Chapter Six

"Finally, there was a doctor who was concerned for human life."

Having gone through several doctors in a short span of time, we now had to search for another pediatrician for Lindsay. I thought that I could go back to Ann Arbor and see Dr. Schmickel—at least he was knowledgeable about MSS and had a warm demeanor. I called him and told him about the difficulties I'd had with several pediatricians. He believed, however, that Lindsay needed a doctor closer to home and that it would not be in her best interest to travel to Ann Arbor. He recommended a doctor at Henry Ford Hospital, the top geneticist in the Detroit area. So I made an appointment and took Lindsay in for an examination. I learned, yet again, that most people in the medical community did not have a clue about MSS.

On one of our visits, Dr. Black brought his residents into the examination room. I happened to be pregnant with Todd, my second child, and an inexperienced resident opened his mouth too soon. He looked at Lindsay, then looked at me and said, "I'm sure you're hoping this won't happen again." My faith in the medical community was all but gone by then.

The conclusion to this appointment? Lindsay was a noisy breather. Dr. Black recommended that she see the Ear, Nose, and Throat specialist, Dr. Glass. I made an appointment and we returned a week later.

After I spoke to Dr. Glass about Lindsay's condition, he determined that she had stridor, or floppy epiglottis, as had been previously suspected. Nothing was done.

In the ensuing months, we continued to visit Henry Ford Hospital for checkups. At one year, Lindsay weighed only 13 pounds, yet there was no medical intervention on her behalf. Lindsay often fell asleep in her high chair while I tried to feed her and had difficulty getting up in the morning and after naps. When her lips took on a bluish cast we immediately called Dr. Black. It was a Saturday. He recommended that she be brought in on Monday and, despite my concerns, I accepted the advice.

Early Monday morning Lindsay was seen at Henry Ford Hospital and, after a cursory examination, the doctor concluded she had low albumin (sugar level) and should be admitted to the hospital for observation. I was seven months pregnant and now Lindsay was in the hospital— what else could go wrong? The anxiety I felt was overwhelming, and I knew that my unborn child, Todd, felt it, too. It seemed like he was going to pop right out of me. I stayed overnight and slept by Lindsay's side. Todd was kicking all night! I had to do everything within my grasp to remain calm for both of them.

Dr. Black made no recommendations about Lindsay's current condition. That's when Dr. Benn Gilmore arrived on the scene. Dr. Gilmore was the new ENT at Henry Ford, replacing Dr. Glass. He was young and had just moved from California. Dr. Gilmore explained that Lindsay's airway was slowly closing and that was the reason she was having breathing difficulties. It was obvious to him when he walked into Lindsay's room and heard her noisy respirations that she was in need of emergency surgery. He explained the nature of a tracheotomy, which was to cut an opening in the trachea and place a tracheostomy tube in the opening that would be secured to the neck with ties. The tube would have to be suctioned frequently to ensure that secretions weren't entering Lindsay's lungs. Hearing this made me feel as if I was an alien on Mars. This was definitely unknown territory. Then Dr. Gilmore said that without this intervention death was imminent—

and I was instantly back down to earth and nodding my approval.

The procedure proved to be a success. I couldn't believe all of the tubes and wires coming out of little Lindsay' body when she was in recovery. This surgery was God sent. I believe it was divine intervention that Dr. Gilmore came back to Michigan to save my daughter. Finally, there was a doctor who was truly committed and concerned for human life, no matter what the patient's condition. Lindsay was fortunate, indeed.

Immediately, we felt a strong bond with Benn Gilmore and are still close to this day. Mary Lynn Harrison and Debbie Hall were Lindsay's primary nurses. They explained the workings of the trach, and they took extraordinary care of Lindsay. She began to thrive almost immediately once she could breathe. It seemed so simple, yet other doctors had been unwilling to intervene. In retrospect, I assume they read the sparse literature and used it as self-fulfilling prophecy—they didn't recommend intervention because they were going to let Lindsay die like the other children with MSS.

After Lindsay's surgery, I no longer had to consult with Dr. Black. I was grateful that Lindsay was in the care of such highly skilled people, and that Dr. Gilmore was on a course to ensure she would have the healthy life she deserved. Lindsay began to gain weight and to sit up. She had a smile that was beyond comprehension. Once again, it was the look she had at birth; the twinkle in her eyes that said, "I'm here to stay." Lindsay was in the hospital for nine weeks and I spent my days by her side. Most evenings I was there as well, until the time she seemed strong enough and I knew that I could go home and sleep.

Family members and friends continually visited the hospital and were very supportive. Immediate family members even learned how to care for Lindsay's tracheotomy. Dr. Gilmore was of the school that others needed to learn about tracheostomy care; otherwise, socialization skills would be deeply hampered. He was so insightful. I couldn't think about anything else at the time, but he was definitely right. I would not be able to do anything by myself if there was no help. My sister, Gayle, her husband, Bernie; my brother, Alan, and his wife, Norma; and brother-in-law and sister-in-law, Mark and Harriet, took on this great responsibility. They all came to the hospital to learn the proper skills in order to care for Lindsay. Mary Lynn and Debbie were skilled teachers and were very patient. For three years, everyone managed to help out whenever the situation arose. They were all loving, kind, and completely supportive. They put aside their own personal schedules to help with Lindsay, and for this I will forever be grateful.

As a matter of fact, Mary Lynn and I became very close friends. She would babysit for Lindsay and Todd, and her husband, Mike, usually came along as well. They even stayed for two long weekends when the kids were quite small. Mary Lynn and Mike were still newlyweds and this certainly gave them a preview of family life. We have celebrated life's milestones together throughout the years. I don't think I would have ever left the kids without knowing Mary Lynn's expert care was readily available. She opened the door for well deserved respite.

The culminating step in the process of taking Lindsay home was a sleepover at Henry Ford Hospital. It wasn't the regular sleepover to keep an eye on her; it was a full 24-hour unsupervised day spent caring for Lindsay with her trach while using the portable suction machine. Whenever Lindsay sounded congested, I would suction her tube to ensure it was clear. All this was done under the careful watch of the medical community. I brought her stroller to the hospital and we would go to the gift shop, and then outside to look at the gardens. Then when all parties involved agreed that the criteria had been met, we left for home.

There was still unfinished business to attend to at Henry Ford Hospital, however, and that was to approach Dr. Black. After nine weeks in the Pediatric Intensive Care Unit—with Lindsay weighing 18 pounds and prospering—it was time to address Lindsay's care, or lack thereof, while under his charge. I made an appointment to speak to Dr. Black in his office. I told him that he'd been lackadaisical in his care for Lindsay and that her diagnosis upon entering the hospital was totally bizarre and didn't apply to her current respiratory failure. He was completely insulted with the use of the word "lackadaisical," as if it tore at his very soul. Dr. Black could not believe that I had the nerve to say he was remiss in his actions when dealing with Lindsay. He proclaimed that he cared for all types of children with genetic problems and that he dedicated his life to the betterment and well-being of all children. I'm sure he truly believed that; and I'm sure that his expertise had been beneficial to many children. However, in Lindsay's case, he'd been ineffective. He did not accept Lindsay as "salvageable." But this was *my* child, *her* life, and all of his education and hard work meant nothing to me because I nearly lost Lindsay. That was unforgivable.

As a matter of fact, several years later, I brought a lawsuit against both Dr. Black and Dr. Glass. Their apathy had continued to gnaw at me and this felt like the proper avenue to pursue—who knows how many other parents had felt the same way about their children's treatment but hadn't spoken up? I wrote out an entire case history; records were obtained, and the lawsuit was put in motion. I suppose an apology would have sufficed, but Dr. Black was too proud to admit his mistake. I met with my attorneys many times and they seemed to feel that the lawsuit centered around negligence. Lindsay would have fared much better with a tracheotomy earlier in her life, they believed, and her impairments might have been minimized if she had an open airway to breathe through. They also felt that Lindsay suffered from carbon dioxide narcosis, which meant that she was keeping the CO_2 in her lungs due to the compromised airway.

After many months of collaboration with the attorneys, the case was filed. Unfortunately, it was concluded that there was "no standard of care" in place for children with MSS. I was absolutely bewildered by this conclusion. It basically meant that since there were so few people with this condition, there was no standard diagnostic course to follow. It was "OK" to do nothing and possibly let someone die, or to live with further complications. My daughter was devalued. I was utterly disappointed, but at least Dr. Black knew that his "lackadaisical" care of Lindsay would not be excused so easily.

"There was no test to see if my next child would have MSS."

In preparation for child number two, I continued to see Dr. Stern. He was back in his practice and healthy after a heart attack, so I decided to give it another shot. At the time, he believed in hypnotizing his patients so they could deliver with less pain. I was all for it, since Lamaze didn't work the first time. Dr. Stern showed me how to concentrate on his voice and visualize his words. He would speak softly and slowly, putting me under a hypnotic spell in his office. It worked! I was totally in another time and space when I listened to his voice. With this success, he recommended we use this technique while in labor with Todd.

I know he was very concerned about delivering a healthy child, but once again another insensitive comment was made by someone in the medical community. During a routine examination I gave Dr. Stern an update on Lindsay and he said, "She will never make it." Well, that was certainly reassuring to a woman expecting her second child! Did he have a direct pipeline to God? (I'm sure he felt he did.)

We proceeded with this unorthodox delivery preparation and, when it was time for Todd to enter this world, I was put into a hypnotic trance. My sister, Gayle, was in the labor room with me as Neil was out of town on business again. Things were going well and I definitely was feeling no pain. Todd, however, wasn't going anywhere. He was too comfortable—and he was also breach. I needed a C-section.

The hypnosis and my euphoria came to a screeching halt. Now I was in transition and experienced excruciating pain. I could hardly wait for the spinal to take effect. Gayle held my hand as I went into the delivery room and was prepped. Dr. Stern asked, "Are we ready?" Gayle put her hands over her face as the incision was made. The thought of blood and the surgical knife made her queasy. I had to ask her if everything was OK. Then Todd arrived and once again all I wanted to know was if he had five fingers, five toes ... and was he healthy? What I was basically asking, however, was, "Does he have MSS?"

I knew that I was looking at a miracle. You see, there was no test to check whether my next child would have MSS. I became pregnant with Todd when Lindsay was just seven months old. Back then, amniocentesis was available only to detect Down syndrome and Spina Bifida. I had this test and all the results came out normal—but there was no guarantee that MSS wouldn't strike again. In all of the literature I'd read—and there wasn't much—there were no reported repeat occurrences in any family who had a child born with MSS. Nevertheless, my anxiety refused to abate and I spent nine months praying for another miracle. Not a day went by that I didn't ask God to protect my unborn child from any and all birth defects. I also had one other request: I could not imagine having another daughter. Even though Lindsay was an infant and I didn't know what her capabilities would be, I could not stand to see her passed by. It would be extremely difficult to watch a younger daughter live life to its fullest while Lindsay struggled. I know this was selfish, but I still prayed, and God was very generous.

Ultimately, my next three children, Todd, Chad, and Eli were born healthy and they were perfect in every way. I experienced the joy of watching healthy boys progress toward life's milestones. No simple act went unnoticed, every smile or movement was held in awe. Rolling over, crawling, and walking were all glorious and I was present to revel in these amazing aspects of childhood development. I took nothing for granted. I knew that this was an enormous blessing. These beautiful baby boys completed me and made it possible to move forward.

When Lindsay and Todd were very young I received a letter in the mail from my mother-in-law, Ethel Weiner. I still have the original envelope and its contents; it was postmarked 1980. I opened it with trepidation, wondering what could be inside—an invitation, perhaps? Why else would she send me a letter when they lived just two streets away? It was an article from the syndicated columnist Erma Bombeck and the subject was handicapped children. Of course, I read it and cried. Did Erma Bombeck know me? She certainly had an affinity for the subject at hand.

The article was titled "The child has his own world." She begins by asserting that "most women become mothers by accident, some by chance and a few by social pressures and a couple by habit." She continues the discussion with statistics concerning the number of children born with impairments. Basically she asks her audience if they are aware of God's vision in selecting mothers for these children. The article paints a picture of God thoughtfully choosing parents for healthy children. He then asks an angel to deliver a handicapped child to an expecting mother. The angel is quite surprised. "Why this one, God? She's so happy." In the course of their discussion God replies to the angel and says "Could I give a handicapped child a mother who does not know laughter? That would be cruel."

It appeared that Erma Bombeck was privy to inside information about the personality and lifestyle of mothers of handicapped children. Did she research and write a case study? Was there a similar situation in her family? Or were her observations prompted by great intuition about a subject that most did not discuss openly during that time period? Erma revealed God's intentions with wit and spot on insight. As the angel listened intently, God discussed the importance of patience, independence, and selfishness. It was explained that a mother of a handicapped child must be able to continue with her life and do things away from her child every once in a while. The notion of "drowning in a sea of self pity and despair" was highlighted. God proclaimed to the angel the absolute necessity of a balanced lifestyle; otherwise the mother would not be able to do her best for the child and the rest of her family.

The beauty of the article is revealed when God tells the angel about the special moments he will grant these mothers. He states that he will enable mothers to enjoy the splendor of their child's progress in life no matter how minute. Even though these moments may seem trivial to women who have healthy children, a mother of a handicapped child will innately understand the miracle of the moment.

As the article concludes, God is also arming mothers of handicapped children with vision about the cruelties of the world, its tragedies and sadness. He states that these special women who have special children will be able to rise above the insanity of the world in order to move forward in life. As God finishes his discussion with the angel he states, "She will never be alone. I will be at her side every minute of every day of her life, because she is doing my work as surely as she is here by my side."

This column resonated in me for many years and after a while I tucked it away in a notebook. Erma Bombeck's words had power and they also soothed. Once I unearthed these pearls of wisdom several years later, I realized how many of her insights were true. It's no wonder that her words left the confines of her small garage, where she began her career, to linger in the hearts of so many loyal readers. Erma knew life and human nature and the combination was explosive.

Chapter Seven

"I had so many 'what if' questions, they were enough to make any mother depressed."

When I was a teenager, I carefully thought about what I wanted to do with my life. I was a planner and didn't like to deviate from the course. I always wanted to be a teacher and my mother was right there to tell Gayle and me that teaching was a great profession for women. She had wanted to be a gym teacher, but her mother didn't have the money to send her to college. So my mother went to work at a local department store in Akron, Ohio and her dreams were realized when both Gayle and I graduated with teaching certificates. She definitely lived vicariously through our experiences. Since Gayle graduated in three years, I thought that I would do the same. (After all, if she could accomplish this feat then so could I.)

I planned out every detail and knew precisely what classes to take in order to graduate early. I attended summer school and loaded up on the classes. I made plans concerning finances and I also thought about the best time to get married, buy a house and, yes, have children. It all seems quite bizarre now.

My plans all seemed to go according to schedule until Lindsay arrived and showed me that even the best laid plans can often go astray. I never took into account that something—or someone—could alter my course. Lindsay showed me that a worthy and noble life is one that is filled with patience and understanding; and in order to be a complete person one has to give without thought of reward. Lindsay opened the door to possibilities that I could never have imagined. I truly learned that long term plans are for the foolhardy since one has to frequently recalculate, responding to life's unexpected challenges.

One plan did work well for me, however. Marty Levinson, a close friend and neighbor, was going to be in the delivery room to welcome and examine Chad when he was born in 1984 and Eli, who was born in1988. Marty was a pediatrician who worked at Sinai Hospital, and he agreed to assist in the delivery room. He was my security blanket and I did not have to deal with anyone else but him after the delivery. Just knowing he cared enough to be there was quite a comfort. After all, how many women have their pediatrician in the delivery room? It was great. Chad and Eli were both delivered by Caesarian section, without a glitch, and after they were cleaned up, Marty began his work. He performed all of the preliminary newborn tests and gave each a passing grade.

I met Marty through his wife, Elise, when our children were about two years old. Josh, their firstborn, has Williams Syndrome. I had never heard of this disorder. There are specific characteristics associated with this condition and they were on a learning curve, just like me. The encouraging part for them was that Josh's condition was not as rare as Lindsay's. They could actually research it and attend educational seminars that proved beneficial.

Lindsay and Josh were in an early intervention program together. When it's determined that a child needs special services due to a birth disorder, programs can begin as early as three months of age. Lindsay received services in our home until she could comfortably attend occupational and physical therapy at a local school. That is when I met Elise.

We were naturally drawn to each other. Our children were about the same age and so were we. As Elise and I forged a relationship at our children's program, we took comfort in being able to share our struggles and concerns. There was a support group in this program and it was good to have connections in a disconnected world.

We realized that Lindsay and Josh were both seen by Chris Gram, a visiting teacher for the three and under crowd from the P.O.H.I. (Physically or Otherwise Health Impaired) program in our school district. Chris visited our homes twice a week to provide the children with essential exercises to help promote their fine and gross motor skills. Even though I was anxious regarding the therapy, it turned out to be quite beneficial for Lindsay.

Chris had a laid-back personality. She was good with Lindsay and I could talk to her about Lindsay's condition, which was still a relatively fresh topic. I was in the beginning stages of trying to understand a baffling syndrome and Chris was not only adept in her profession, she was a good sounding board as well. She had the capacity to listen and not judge. Her visits were quite therapeutic for me. Chris was the first professional to work with Lindsay, and I could implicitly trust her.

I was in unexplored territory and I needed a capable guide. Through this program I started to become familiar with the world of physical and occupational therapy. I didn't realize that there were so many sub-areas connected to these fields. I had to investigate each growth opportunity for Lindsay, and Chris helped immensely in this capacity.

Her daughter, Megan, was disabled, and slowly Chris began to tell me about her challenges. She never did so in order to help alleviate my pain; rather, Chris integrated various situations concerning Megan into our conversations. For example, when I discussed concerns about Lindsay not achieving milestones, Chris told a story about a church experience she had. Her family was seated in the pews listening to the Sunday service when she viewed a young girl across the aisle holding a doll. This girl was approximately the same age as Megan and she was undressing and dressing her doll. There was nothing unusual about the scene—most girls delight in making their dolls look "just so." But Chris fixated on the natural rhythm of the girl's motions and how easily she could complete the task. Of course, this reminded Chris that her daughter would have had great difficulty with such an endeavor. The things that people take for granted are the very things mothers of disabled children marvel at.   I understood completely.

I had so many "what if" questions. What if Lindsay declines? What if her breathing problems return? What if I find her unresponsive? What if she never walks, talks, and is unable to care for herself? These questions were enough to make any mother depressed. Since depression was not a part of my demeanor, however, I had to stop torturing myself and let life happen. I resolved that I would deal with the fallout later. Benn Gilmore used to tell me that Lindsay was writing the book on MSS and her story would have a different outcome than those in the past.   I savored those words.

"Along with all the many frightening characteristics of MSS, there was also the element of advanced bone age."

After so many negative encounters with doctors, it was refreshing to have Marty as Lindsay's pediatrician. He treated her with respect and was always available for my seemingly endless questions. Marty was now her advocate, just like Benn Gilmore. I finally felt a sense of relief and even a nice comfort level because of these two men.

It was reassuring to me that all of the children loved to go to Marty's office. He was not a traditional white coat doctor. (There's nothing more daunting than a white coat marching toward a child.) To the contrary, Marty sported colorful shirts, sometimes decorated with Disney characters or flowers. They were warm and inviting. And Marty never wore a tie either, but he did wear the most interesting socks. (Children pick up on these things.) He always had a quick wit and an inviting disposition.

Certainly it's not the exterior that makes the man; it was his dedication that was key to his success. I could call him at any time of day or night concerning a medical issue with the kids and he would always return my calls. His accessibility was amazing and he never made me feel that I was annoying. And for that reason, Todd, Chad, and Eli enjoyed going to his office, and Lindsay always had a smile when he entered the room. They knew he cared. Waiting for their appointments, they would cruise down the hall on roller chairs and enjoy themselves until it was their turn. Of course, this activity was only tolerated when it was the end of the day and the rest of the patients had checked out. Marty took excellent care of my children and everyone else's. His reputation in the community is held in the highest regard. Lindsay was finally in luck with such a compassionate and dedicated physician.

As the years marched on, I took solace in the fact that these two professionals were only a phone call away. I could discuss the various problems that Lindsay's condition presented and there would always be contemplation followed by action.

Along with all of the many frightening characteristics of MSS, there was also the element of advanced bone age. Benn and I discussed the idea of making an appointment with an endocrinologist at Henry Ford Hospital. We also wanted to maximize Lindsay's growth potential, since advanced bone age meant that Lindsay would stop growing at an early age. So I made the appointment and the doctor seemed quite interested in testing Lindsay to see if there was anything he could do to slow body hair growth and possibly help with Lindsay's short stature. Blood was taken and Dr. Klein said that he would study the problem and get back to me when he had the results. I felt that he was genuinely concerned and would research any and all ideas.

Wow, my barometer was totally wrong.

After several weeks I finally received a letter in the mail from the department of endocrinology at Henry Ford Hospital. I tentatively opened it and read a short, concise letter. In its brevity the good doctor stated: "Lindsay's bone age on 4-20-82 was 6 years 10 months. She was 36 months at that time and this compares with a bone age of 3 years 6 months when she was 9 months and another of 5 years 6 months when she was 23 months. Unfortunately, we have no way of altering the rapid progression of her bone age." That was it—batta boom, batta bing—there was no commentary about her blood work or hirsutism (hair growth). I guess I was hoping for too much.

Nonetheless, I was awestruck. Dr. Klein knew how desperately I was searching for some type of remedy and all he could do with the information was to write me a short, cold, statistical letter. I already knew her bone age at these various points in time, and I certainly didn't need them repeated. At the very least he should have called me to explain the outcome, or lack thereof. This insensitivity outraged me and I don't think that I was over reacting. Where was the human element? I decided that the next time I had to take Lindsay to see Benn Gilmore for a checkup I would casually stroll over to Dr. Klein's office and confront him about his callous behavior.

I waited two weeks. I had gone over the scenario many times in my head. I was ready. Upon arriving at Henry Ford Hospital I approached the central kiosk to check in for Lindsay's appointment. There was a man standing in front of us and when he was finished, he turned around and glanced down at Lindsay. Then he looked at me and said, "They can't all be normal." His comment was like a slap across the face. I wasn't ready for that; are you ever? What the hell is wrong with people? I certainly didn't need this distraction before my encounter with the good doctor.

Lindsay and I took the elevator to the fifth floor and then I took her out of her stroller. I asked the receptionist if Dr. Klein was in his office or seeing patients. I was told that she would let him know I wanted to speak with him. As I recollect, I did not wait to be called in; I simply walked past the receptionist and strolled into his office. All the while I was ignoring the pleas of, "You must wait like everyone else! You can't go in there!" But I did, and with a vengeance.

I do believe that there was a greeting somewhere in my introduction and I definitely reviewed our past visit. Dr. Klein sat behind his desk and simply listened to my complaint. I held his letter in my hand and, with clarity, told him how offended I was that he sent such a cold letter. I stated that he should have called and I was surprised that he lacked the insight to communicate with me on a personal level. I continued saying that Lindsay's situation was not the norm and there should have been more sensitivity. Dr. Klein's response still lingers in my head. He took a few seconds to reply and then said, "Well stated." There was neither apology nor regret in his voice. I turned on my heels and Lindsay and I walked out of his office.

Chapter Eight

"I told my mother I needed positive thoughts only."

Bob, Marian, Sam, and Ethel were all wonderful grandparents. (Lou and Claire, my second husband, Jeffrey's, parents, were also caring and attentive with Lindsay.) At the onset, they all suspected that something was amiss with Lindsay, but they handled themselves well, asked a lot of questions, and accepted the fact that answers were not always available. I recognized they all were quite sad and very concerned.

When my brother, Alan, was 22 years old he worked at Hawthorne Metal in Royal Oak, earning money as a stamping press operator while attending college. My brother was a conscientious employee. One time, however, when he placed the flat metal sheet into the press, it came down on his hands—without him pushing the activation button—and crushed them under the heavy weight of the machine. I can't imagine the excruciating pain Alan must have felt at that moment. After that, all I remember were his heavily bandaged hands and the daily hospital visits. My parents were devastated. My father tried to be encouraging. A few times, he brought a friend to the hospital who had also lost some fingers in an accident. Thanks to those visits, my brother saw that it was possible to recover from such a debilitating accident and actually have a life.

Unfortunately, though Alan eventually recovered from his accident, my mother never did. She lost weight (and believe me, she really did not have much to lose as she was already quite thin). Every time I went shopping with her and she encountered friends, the crying would begin anew as she recounted the horrors of her son's accident. I can't say exactly how many times this occurred, but it seemed like hundreds. I was mortified. I was 13 years old and couldn't comprehend the drama. Certainly I knew that my mother was in pain, but I had no idea about a mother's loss. I simply grew weary of the scene. My brother, on the other hand, was tough. He had many skin grafts to ensure a smoother appearance of the remaining fingers. Alan continued with his daily routine and went to an occupational therapist to learn how to maximize his hand and finger use. He learned to cope, but my mother never did. His perseverance was astonishing, and even though I did not realize it at the time, I was watching a role model.

Alan was engaged when the accident occurred, and shortly afterward got married. The marriage did not last long and I presume that his accident placed a great deal of psychological pressure on both of them. Alan kept his hands behind his back a lot of the time and the trauma of the accident must have been unrelenting. When they filed for divorce a few years later, my mother stepped right back into her crying routine whenever we were in public. I was once again mortified and had to incur the repeated misery of listening to the saga of the failed marriage whenever we met her friends.

I wished that I could just disappear.

So, when Lindsay had that lengthy hospitalization to have her trach implanted, I decided I had to broach the subject with my mother. I told her that I needed positive thoughts only—crying in front of me or Lindsay was absolutely out of the question. She respected my demand and then, consequently, began to cry to my sister. Old habits are tough to kick, but at least I didn't have to endure the torture anymore, though my poor sister Gayle did.

I must say that my mom was a remarkable woman. She was great with Lindsay. Any time I needed her to help out she was there in an instant. And I needed her a lot. My parents were the poster-seniors for the world's best grandparents. They gave unconditional love to Lindsay and my three boys. My mom would take long walks, pulling them in our Little Tikes wagon while meandering through the neighborhood. Everyone knew my parents. And then, when my dad retired from driving a truck for a meat commissary, he began his second job: caring for his grandchildren. They were lovingly known as the "super duo."

Mom and Dad would accompany me to doctor appointments, watch Lindsay when I wanted to meet friends, and even stay overnight. I returned to teaching when Lindsay was 11 and Eli, my youngest, was two and a half years old. I only worked part-time, but I needed their assistance. They were at my house every day to greet the kids upon their return from school. They would give all of the kids a snack and even pick up the car pool if I couldn't make it. (It was difficult to be at three different schools at the same time, plus get Lindsay off her bus.) Todd and Chad would request chicken tenders when they returned from school and Eli always wanted a large ice cream sundae with chocolate syrup. Lindsay had a ten cookie appetizer of Chips Ahoy. (We had actual stock in these cookies, both from the Phillip Morris Company and in our pantry. There were never less than four packages of these delightful morsels on the shelves.)

After snack time, my dad would take Lindsay for a ride. Now, this was no ordinary ride down the street. This was my dad's most important job and he made sure that Lindsay had a good time. Cruising Woodward Avenue was their favorite pastime. The key to the drive was the musical accompaniment. My dad always had tapes of Cab Calloway, Louis Armstrong, and Al Jolson. This ritual of love continued for many years until my dad had to retire from his second and most important job. His health began to fail at age 83 and he grew too weak to take Lindsay on her special rides. My siblings and I now had to care for my dad, and he did not like the role reversal.

At this point my second husband, Jeffrey, started to take over Lindsay's after school care, and my dad slowly stopped coming over. We asked him to visit, but he regretted the fact that he could no longer sustain his special relationship with Lindsay. Knowing my dad, he was saddened; too, that he had a replacement. However, in his sadness he took great comfort in the knowledge that Jeffrey was the person best suited to take his position. All my dad wanted was to know that his angel, Lindsay, was going to be loved and cared for. In Jeffrey, he had found his answer.

Sam and Ethel, my first husband's parents, redefined the traditional role of grandparents. They were not the type to babysit, as they led a very active life. They were constantly on the go. Whether out to the movies, out to eat, or out on the town, Sam and Ethel did not spend much time hanging around their house. As a result, their involvement with the grandchildren revolved around some of their favorite activities. The children loved to go out to eat with them and, of course, I would always come along to help with Lindsay. We all went to the theatre to see children's plays and the special treat was going bowling with grandma and grandpa. (Ethel was a sight to behold on the lanes. She would approach the pins just like Fred Flintstone; small quick steps and on her toes.) And Grandpa Sam always had a good business proposition for the kids. They would scratch his back until he was content and then he would give them each a quarter. It was quite a slick operation.

Jeffrey and I got married on December 20th, 1997. Lou and Claire, Jeffrey's parents, were in their 70s and had their own special routine with the kids. They would come over for dinner, enjoying the bustling activity of a house full of kids. Lou was famous for his corny jokes and everyone listened attentively—even when he repeated the same ones over and over.

Sadly enough, they are all gone now. The last to go was my mother. She spent her final days in a nursing home.

Whenever I visited without Lindsay because she was at school or running errands with Jeffrey, the first words out of my mom's mouth were, "Where's my Lindsay?" I guess I wasn't good enough! When I brought Lindsay, which I did several times a week, my mom would carry on a conversation with her while hardly talking to me. It was a sight to behold, this one-sided conversation. It breaks my heart that so many of the people that Lindsay loved have left us far too soon.

Chapter Nine

"All eyes were on Lindsay as she commenced to strike the first symbol and let the smooth, silky voice resonate throughout the sanctuary."

At the age of 13 Lindsay became a Bat Mitzvah. I was determined that she partake in this rite of passage like everyone else's Jewish daughter. The idea had been marinating in my mind for many years and, as the appropriate time approached, I met with Rabbi Steinger. He told me that he would do whatever was needed in order to make this dream come true. After this initial meeting I spoke to the Rabbi frequently to solidify the plans.

Lindsay had been attending Sunday school classes for special needs children for several years. She truly liked the program and looked forward to this activity. Every Sunday, I would sit outside the room and wait until the hour-long class ended. They basically did fun assignments that centered around different aspects of Judaism, such as coloring picture representations of Torah scenes and cooking holiday treats. I also took Lindsay to Temple quite often since Todd was in Hebrew school at the time. We attended various services to watch the Bar and Bat Mitzvah programs and to learn exactly what was expected.

When Lindsay was given a date for her special event, we contacted Michigan State University to find a specialist in augmentative devices. Lindsay used "The Wolf " and it generated a mechanical voice that definitely sounded like a male; we wondered if it was possible to find a device that sounded like a female. John Eulenberg, Associate Professor and Director of the Artificial Language Laboratory, had assisted many people with this situation. John knew too well the challenges of the disabled. He'd watched as his father, a vibrant public speaker who had loved to converse, contracted Lou Gehrig's disease. It soon became impossible for him to communicate. He died in 1968. However, that was not John's first experience with the disabled. His best friend, who was blind, had used a Braille prayer book at his Bar Mitzvah ceremony. The two young men became determined to work for the elimination of handicap obstructers. And so John set out on the road to M.I.T., then Harvard, and the University of California-San Diego, from which he holds a Ph.D. in computer science and linguistics. It became his passion to help needy individuals find their voices with the use of adaptive equipment. He said that he would be happy to give Lindsay a feminine voice so that she could "recite" her Torah portion.

Lindsay's Bat Mitzvah date was June 5th. The portion of the Torah that coincided with that date was abbreviated so that it fit on a panel that could be activated by Lindsay's touch. There were ten sections for Lindsay to hit with her hand, all of which had the sweet sound of Lindsay's artificial voice.

An article written for *The Jewish News* in 1992 stated:

'Lindsay's Torah portion is from Numbers 3. Her verses include a description of how God, in killing the firstborn of Egypt, spared the firstborn of Israel and claimed them for His own. Lindsay is the firstborn in her family. Here she will be at her bat mitzvah having *lived,*' Dr. Eulenberg says. 'She, too, was spared the death from which many other children (with Marshall-Smith syndrome) have died. And now, she will perform the service, the priestly function of praising God and reading from the Torah.'

The Temple was filled with friends, family, and the usual Saturday congregants. As Lindsay stood behind the *bimah* I knew this special time was God sent. His presence was in the air and felt by everyone. All eyes were on Lindsay as she commenced to strike the first symbol and let the smooth, silky voice resonate throughout the sanctuary. It was amazing to watch as Lindsay hit each of the ten targets and smile because she knew this was her day. The first part was called *Barchu et Adoshem Hamevorach*—the blessing before the reading of the Torah. I, too, felt blessed for this incredible day in Lindsay's life.

Years later, ensconced in my teaching career, I was at parent/teacher conferences at Berkley High School. While waiting for the next parent to come up to my table and discuss their child's progress, I recognized a familiar face. This father had been at Lindsay's Bat Mitzvah, but in a professional capacity. He'd walked up to the *bimah* and handed Lindsay the usual gifts that are presented to the Bar/Bat Mitzvah after the ceremony. His son was in my class and it had been a long time since Lindsay's Bat Mitzvah. Before we began the preliminary sharing of information concerning academics, he paused and reflected back to Lindsay's special day. He confessed that as he presented Lindsay with her gifts that day he was crying, not only during that moment, but throughout the entire service, like many others. I knew those tears oh so well. They were tears of joy and tears of sorrow. I also must think that those tears represent a bit of gratitude for the health of his own children. Watching Lindsay stirs an appreciation for the miracle many take for granted.

"Todd cared about Lindsay's happiness and instilled this sentiment in his younger brothers. I don't believe it was a conscious effort; Todd simply did what came naturally."

Throughout every step of Lindsay's life, her brothers have been by her side. I once read that the siblings of impaired individuals are the most compassionate, understanding, and loving people. Todd, Chad, and Eli definitely fit into this category. Since Todd is just 16½ months younger than Lindsay, they formed a close bond right away. As they were growing up, Lindsay was always at Todd's side. He regarded Lindsay as his sister, not his handicapped sister.

However, one day as we were on our way out of the supermarket, Todd approached me about a comment he'd overheard at the checkout counter. He said, "Mom, that boy behind us said that Lindsay is 'rearted.' What does that mean?" The comment caught me off guard—and cut like a knife as well. I proceeded to explain that the correct pronunciation was "retarded" and that he knew Lindsay's development was slower than others. Todd was probably six years old at the time. He was well aware that Lindsay had a very rare condition. How could I make him understand the implications of Marshall-Smith Syndrome? So, each time it was appropriate, I would point out the facts that he could comprehend. After all, he was a very bright, very perceptive young boy. Todd grew to become quite protective of his sister.

A few years later a similar incident occurred. We were enjoying a fine summer's day at the Huntington Woods pool, splashing around in the shallow end. Todd had brought a friend along, as usual, and everyone seemed to be having fun. I was holding Lindsay while bobbing up and down so she, too, could enjoy an underwater experience. Chad, Eli, and their buddies were also playing. Shortly after, Todd and his friend swam over to me and said hello. Then as quickly as they appeared, they were off. Minutes later, Todd reappeared and told me that his friend said that Lindsay was ugly. I didn't know how to respond to that so I told him to ignore the comment. All the while I was seething on the inside. I couldn't protect him from these ignorant comments and I knew that they must have been very hurtful. Todd, Chad, and Eli would have to navigate this terrain by themselves. That was the last time Todd played with that young boy. Thankfully, he had many other friends who were kind and enjoyed being with Lindsay.

As Todd proceeded through high school and then college, his thoughts were anchored to Lindsay. Even though he had a busy social life, he always made time for his sister. He would drive to the mall with Chad and Eli, and they always took Lindsay, too. If Jeffrey and I needed someone to watch Lindsay so we could go out for an evening alone, Todd would volunteer. Todd cared about Lindsay's happiness and instilled this sentiment in his younger brothers. I don't believe it was a conscious effort; Todd simply did what came naturally.

At 22, after he graduated with a degree in psychology from Wayne State University, Todd decided to go to Israel to study in a Yeshiva for two months. In his last year of college he'd attended a Torah study group at our neighbor's house. Todd also studied with a Rabbi during the week and he wanted to further his Jewish education. Jeffrey and I decided that this trip would be a good graduation gift. As it turns out, it became the gift that kept on giving. He returned after ten months and then went back again for another year. The rest is history; Todd has been in Israel for ten years, and he now has a beautiful wife and three daughters. I know that when he left for Israel he did so with a heavy heart. First of all, he was headed to a strange country by himself and secondly, he was sad to leave for so long. Todd stated that he knew he could embark on this journey because Lindsay would receive all the help she needed from Chad and Eli. As it turned out, he handed over the torch to two very capable young men.

At this point in time, Chad was in his sophomore year of college at Wayne State University and Eli was in the tenth grade at Berkley High School. Chad truly enjoyed taking Lindsay for rides in his car and blasting the music. He loved to see Lindsay move back and forth in her seat to the rhythm of the songs. His car would reverberate as he sang out loud and cruised around the neighborhood. Some might find blasting music a nuisance, but Lindsay beamed with pleasure from this experience. Even now, his absolute favorite activity is driving Lindsay to the Somerset Mall. After some shopping or taking in the sights, they usually head for the food court. Chad orders Lindsay her favorite beverage: a tall glass of Coke. He delights in Lindsay's pleasure as he describes the manner in which she savors her drink. She holds the large cup in her right hand and extends it outward as if she's at a cocktail party sipping on a martini. The visual is delightful.

Chad can always sense when I need some help and he chimes in perfectly to let me know that he will hang out with Lindsay, run some errands, or take her out to eat. Lindsay likes to take Chad's hand and drag him outside for a walk or to sit on the porch. She might reach out for him whenever he enters the room and this is the cue, as if she is saying, "pick me up and spend some time with me." The smile on his face is absolutely beautiful as he acknowledges his sister's request. It's a sight to behold.

When Chad was two years old, Shelley and Jack Jaffe moved into the house next door. They had a son, Brent, who was Chad's age, and they became fast friends—or, more accurately, partners in crime. As they meandered around the neighborhood on their Big Wheels and Little Tikes cars, Lindsay and I would be right next to them; or at least trying to keep up with this dynamic duo. I can still picture them sitting on top of Chad's bunk bed, throwing Goldfish crackers on the floor and laughing hysterically. Lindsay was there, too, but she was with me on the cleaning end of this fiasco, eating her share of Goldfish as I picked up the mess. The boys also enjoyed sitting on the lawn with our dog, Cecil. Lindsay would join in on the fun since Cecil was such a good sport. She would pull his hair in an attempt to pet him. Chad and Brent would loyally help Cecil escape from Lindsay's firm grasp. (They would also come to the rescue when Eli began to ride Cecil like a horse.)

Over time, as Lindsay's arthritis grew more severe, she developed difficulty walking because of the pain. Chad has been there to help us out. He's young, strong, and volunteers to carry Lindsay up the stairs to her bedroom. If the weather is inclement and we're in the car, Chad will come outside and carry Lindsay into the house. Conversely, if Lindsay is stiff and acting like she is standing in cement, Chad will pick her up and take her to a comfortable spot. He does not want to see his sister in pain, and it hurts him to witness her distress.

Chad has paved the way for Eli as well. Eli has grown up knowing that Lindsay faces great challenges. Eli has observed his two role models throughout the years and he intuitively knows what's required of him in this family. When Eli walks in the house he does so with a great deal of gusto. Usually the first thing he blurts out is, "Mina B." This is his pet name for Lindsay and he says it in a high, unmistakable pitch. Lindsay immediately laughs upon hearing this funny sounding name and the tone in which it is delivered. Eli always has a big hug and kiss for his sister. He wears sports caps quite frequently and Lindsay loves to grab them and pitch those caps to the floor. This also causes her to crack up. She will then rub his head affectionately as he sits next to her on the sofa.

As a young boy, Eli was obsessed with watching WWF wrestling matches on television and then reenacting them with his friends. They would drag out an old mattress and a belt that was adorned with the WWF insignia. The belt was bestowed with pride on whoever won the latest match. The boys would create their own style of wrestling and try to carry out interesting moves just like those nuts on television. Even though we told them that the wrestling matches were staged and definitely not real, I do think they still believed in the power of those muscle men. Lindsay enjoyed watching the boys perform their wrestling moves and they liked the audience participation. The entire family would laugh at this ritual of entertainment. And as each of Eli's friends walked through the front door they, too, would be sure to seek out Lindsay. Without knowing it, Todd, Chad, and Eli showed their friends that Lindsay was a valuable person who was capable of interaction with others, even though she had no language skills. These friends knew that the reach of her hand and the smile on her face were enough. And, if they were lucky, Lindsay would make some of her happy sounds for them.

In middle school, Eli wrote a report about his sister and explained, in laymen's terms, the nuances of Lindsay's condition. There were plenty of pictures to accompany the project. He was careful to mention all of the things his sister could do instead of dwelling on the negatives. Since

Lindsay was always a visible force in his school and the community, most people were familiar with his subject. I recall his teacher commenting that she had witnessed the love and affection that Eli bestowed upon his sister when she came to watch his basketball games. She said that she was truly touched and that Eli had given a valuable lesson to his peers. This type of behavior did not go unnoticed by his friends. Whenever we were in the stands at Berkley High School or at another school for a sporting event, his friends always made it a point to come by our seats to say hello and sit for a while with Lindsay. Some would put an arm around her and others would plant a kiss on her cheek. Lindsay has definitely affected many souls.

Trying to imagine my sons' feelings about Lindsay has always been difficult. I know the sadness and the joy from a mother's perspective; but from their view? Now that is a challenge. I cannot walk in their shoes, nor can I make the situation any different. I don't think I would have handled this lifelong sense of obligation as generously as they have done thus far. They are remarkable young men and I am very proud of them. However, I am always aware of the fact that they must carve out their own paths in life. I also know there must have been times when they have felt discouraged, embarrassed, or simply wondered about the family dynamics had Lindsay been born an average, healthy person. All of this pondering reminded me of a poem I enjoyed when I was in college.

The Prophet, by Kahlil Gibran, a poem entitled "On Children" best expresses my sentiments. I would read this book forward and backward to find direction, solace and comfort. I never imagined that one day I would reflect upon it again for its total and complete honesty as applied to my own life. In this poem, Gibran discusses the notion of children being sent forth in life like "living arrows." And parents are the archers with their bent bows—ready to help their children move forward. He was really talking about releasing your children—letting them go once they are capable of being on their own. Gibran stated "Your children are not your children. They are the sons and daughters of Life longing for itself." He knew that parents have to relinquish their grip—their control. Gibran went on to say that, as parents, we have dreams for our children. However, they too have dreams of their own and this must be respected. We also cannot try to mold our children to be like us. Parents must encourage and inspire. Gibran then stated that our children's "souls dwell in the house of tomorrow." So they must create their future and make their own decisions.

Chapter Ten

"Jeffrey was well aware that he had taken on an incredible task—a journey that would be fulfilling as well as frustrating."

When Jeffrey and I started dating in 1994, his parents and friends thought he was crazy. They asked him why he wanted to date a woman with four children, one of whom was severely impaired. They all thought he was out of his mind. And I'm sure, at times, he probably thought he was, too. Yet, we had a deep connection from our high school and college days. Jeffrey was my best friend and I lost that bond many years ago. Our relationship began to blossom again as if time had never passed. Nearly twenty years had slipped away, but it felt as if we were back at Oak Park High. (Jeffrey is a remarkable man. His love for me never wavered for 20 years—throughout my first marriage and after the divorce.) I couldn't wait to see him, to talk to him, and spend as much time with him as possible. All I kept thinking was, "I've got my best friend back." Jeffrey and I would meet for lunch, go to movies, or just hang out and talk for hours.

Several months into the relationship we decided it was time for the children to meet him. They were well aware that their mother was dating "Jeffrey Markowitz" and now they were ready to put a face to the name. At the time Eli was 6, Chad was 9, Todd was 14, and Lindsay was 15. What a handful!

Jeffrey entered the scene with style and grace. However, I'm sure he was shaking in his boots. He gained their confidence by playing with them whenever he was around. He would go outside to play catch or toss around the football. They enjoyed Jeffrey's company. He forged a relationship with the kids simply by being available, and by showing them how to treat a woman—their mother. They were glad to know that I was finally happy.

The kids were in awe of this man who cooked meals, helped with the clean up after dinner, and sat with them to complete homework assignments. (A remarkable contrast.) When report card time rolled around, Jeffrey would joke and ask "What grade did I get?" And then the boys once stated, "Mom, Jeffrey treats you like a queen." My response was that this is the way a man and woman should interact. I told them that their mother was not on a throne, she was simply loved.

After three and a half years of developing a solid relationship with me and the children, we decided to get married. I'm sure his family and friends still thought that he was dazed and confused. Regardless, we set the date and made all of the plans. I must say that it was one of the happiest days of my life. Lindsay, Todd, Chad, and Eli walked down the aisle and they were elated. What could be better than having your children witness your wedding day?

Jeffrey loved the boys and Lindsay from the onset. He was well aware that he had taken on an incredible task, a journey that would be fulfilling and frustrating. Yet he slid into the role of father easily. Jeffrey finally had a family and I had a partner who was willing to share in my life's adventure.

Todd, Chad, and Eli knew how much Jeffrey loved Lindsay. This was very important to them. It also amazed Jeffrey that he could so easily become attached to a child with severe impairments. After all, he had never spent any time with an individual who had special needs. He brought out the best in Lindsay. Since she could not talk, except for a few words, she would begin to vocalize sounds whenever Jeffrey entered a room. Lindsay spoke to him in her own language and he knew how to communicate with her. She would caress his bald head and give him "love smacks" as a sign of affection. They would play and cuddle for hours. Lindsay had a blast climbing all over him.

As time progressed, Jeffrey began to take Lindsay to physical therapy, doctor appointments, shopping, and out to restaurants by himself. We became a team in the morning as well, getting Lindsay ready for school and onto the bus.

As a matter of fact, Jeffrey takes care of Lindsay's personal needs as well. He does not hesitate to assist her in the bathroom. Lindsay requires help with pulling her pants down and then up when using the toilet. She also needs guidance to sit on the toilet. And even more help is required when Lindsay has her period. Jeffrey has definitely learned the nuances of feminine hygiene products. There are also occasions when Lindsay will have accidents and Jeffrey cleans her up, changes her underwear and clothes, and makes sure she is comfortable. How many men would take on this challenge? Simply put, Jeffrey is amazing.

Chapter Eleven

"She can't read or write but she is aware of what is going on in her world and she can interact with others—that is, when she feels like it."

Lindsay needs assistance in every facet of her life. From the minute she wakes up in the morning until she goes to bed at night, someone has to be with her. She has also become a night owl and does not maintain regular sleep habits. Until Lindsay was 15 she slept like a rock. The house could be in an uproar and she would not stir. Then the tables completely turned. After she stopped taking Tegretol for a seizure disorder she'd developed at age six, she began to wake up in the night and cry out. I was glad that she no longer exhibited seizure tendencies since these took on the form of a breathing disorder—a problem that compounded existing respiratory issues with MSS—but the sleep-interrupted nights were not easy to deal with. At first either Jeffrey or I would go into Lindsay's bedroom and reassure her and she would go back to sleep. As time went on, however, she awoke more frequently and we eventually found ourselves falling asleep in her room or bringing her to our bed. We know she just wants company. (We have concluded that Lindsay would very much enjoy having a boyfriend.)

We definitely have our daily routine down pat: wake up, go to the bathroom, brush Lindsay's teeth, style her hair, wash her face, get her dressed, and make the slow descent down the stairs into the kitchen to have breakfast. Lindsay loves cereal and some of her all time favorites are Fruit

Loops, Apple Jacks, Honey Nut Cheerios, and Crispix. Lindsay will let us know her basic needs by shaking her head yes or no to simple questions. She will also reach for items she wants or take our hands and walk us to her desired destination.

At lunch or dinner, all food must be cut into bite-size pieces. Pudding, yogurt, cereal, ice cream, and basically all soft foods are not a problem and are easily consumed. She can use a spoon quite well, but we must supervise in order to assure that she does not place too much food in her mouth; and we must constantly be mindful of dripping and wiping her mouth. She usually can manage quite well, but vigilance deters spills on her clothing or the floor. (When Lindsay had her trach all food had to be pureed so that she would not aspirate anything into her lungs. That was a bit tricky.)

Lindsay can be Houdini-like at the dinner table. I usually have a napkin under her plate that extends to her clothing to soak up minor spills. Well, Lindsay has been known to grab that napkin, sometimes without causing the plate to move, but often by dumping some of the food. At other times she grips the plate and tosses it. (I suppose she's entitled to break a few like anyone else.) She definitely has her moods. However, when she falls into a particularly bad mood during a meal, we have learned to take precautions.

When Lindsay was small I laminated picture cards of colors, cars, the school bus, food, relatives, and everything else of relevance in her life. I would then ask her to place her hand on a particular picture and this let me know that she was learning about the world around her. Lindsay received her first communication device when she was six years old. It was called The Wolf; a small machine about the size of a laptop. There was a frame around it with four spaces to insert pictures. When a particular item was touched—or in Lindsay's case, knocked with her knuckles—an automated voice would speak her selection. "I want Apple Jacks," was a frequent sound. Lindsay was quite adept at using The Wolf. However, it soon became apparent that Lindsay could reply with a head shake for yes or no responses to questions faster than I could change the pictures on the communication board. It was more practical to simply ask her the questions and wait for an answer.

Lindsay is a woman on a mission. She loves to be active and we are on the move all the time. She definitely knows what she wants, and if she does not feel like responding she will lower her head and act coy. It's a great tactic to avoid people and I've seen her do this hundreds of times. This coyness plays into testing situations at school. Every three years while attending public school programs, children receiving special services have to take a psychological test. These tests determine appropriate levels of functioning for cognition, gross motor, and fine motor. Her scores are always low and this is naturally quite depressing. It's enough to make me cry when I hear her level of functioning as compared to a healthy individual. However, throughout the years I have learned that even though the scores on these tests reveal that Lindsay is severely multiply impaired, the fact that she can communicate with us and let her needs be known is satisfying enough. She can't read or write but she is aware of what is going on in her world and she can interact with others—when she feels like it. There is nothing more comforting than when she rubs my arm affectionately or places her hand in mine. And when Lindsay smiles it melts my soul. She has a twinkle in her eyes when she is in a glorious mood and words can't describe just how good this makes me feel. Lindsay chirping, happy sounds let us know that all is well.

For the most part, Lindsay is a very happy and social young lady, but her demeanor can change dramatically. When she is irritable, she has a tendency to let us know, big time. She might pull my hair or turn her sweet love nibbles into outright bites. Lindsay delivers her anger swiftly and without warning. We call these, jokingly, "shark attacks." Fortunately, such times are short lived and Lindsay almost immediately wants to make up. It's quite difficult to resist her gentle touch at those moments.

The most disturbing thing Lindsay will do out of anger is bang her head on the kitchen table for a special effect. The sound is frightening. When Lindsay was learning to walk she took quite a few spills and landed on her head. Several times she received stitches and, as a result, there is a lot of scar tissue on her scalp. And that is the exact area that Lindsay targets. Fortunately, she's never caused an injury to herself from this action. Lindsay must have the hardest head in town. I believe this is her way of venting—an outlet for all of her frustrations—since she can't stamp her feet or yell obscenities.

Overall, I try to keep in tune with Lindsay's moods and feelings. I try to imagine how I might feel in her situation, attempting to look at things from her perspective—Lindsay's view from four foot two. While helping her to get dressed I am always cognizant of her comfort. When pulling up her pants or putting on tights, I'm careful with the fit. Also, underwear should be smooth and in place so as not to crawl up her tush. I make sure that her socks are not bunched up, around or in her toes, and that shoes fit comfortably. The laces should never be pulled too tight and the tongue of the shoe should be in place and not sliding back; which could be painful. If a shirt needs to be tucked into her pants or skirt, I smooth it out so that it won't annoy her. Pockets are another problem area. If they are crunched up and not in place this could also be a source of irritation. By far the biggest factor in clothing is shortening the arms of shirts, sweaters, and jackets, and adjusting the length of pants and skirts. Due to Lindsay's short stature, practically every item needs attention. I also have to be certain that clothing is appropriate for her age and, at times, this is a true test, given her size. Lindsay wears children's or teens clothing and her feet are quite small as well. She wears a size one and a half shoe. I am always hunting for cute yet sophisticated clothing. Luckily, we both love to shop.

When choosing a car to lease or buy, Lindsay is the first factor I consider. Since she is petite, I need a car that will accommodate her needs. Some seats are too low and she can't look out of the window. Comfortable seats are also a consideration. Lindsay enjoys being on the road, so we take long rides listening to the radio or an audio book. A hatchback is also a must because of the space it provides for her wheelchair. Running boards were helpful at a time when Lindsay could maneuver them. She would step on the board and then, with assistance, get in to the car. When her arthritis kicked in with a vengeance, however, she had to be lifted and placed into her seat. Lindsay is a front seat lady because it affords the best views. (The passenger seat airbag must be turned off.)

Another area of consideration is styling Lindsay's hair. She has thick, beautiful, short dark hair. I let it grow out once and there was just so much hair everywhere. (I'm talking about hair that had a mind of its own and Lindsay looked like a wild woman. It was a throwback to the crazy hairstyles of the 70s.) So after several years of trying to tame that hair, it was cut into a classic manageable style.

When Lindsay was 18 years old I began to notice gray hairs. I was not surprised, as this had occurred with me as well. I had long hair as a teenager and when I, too, was 18 gray hairs began to appear. Eventually there were two long streaks of gray on each side of my part. What an attractive sight! People even asked me if I had my hair colored to achieve this effect. In my mid-twenties I joined forces with the salon, and hair color became my mainstay —no more gray for me. Thus, when Lindsay's hair began to take on the salt and pepper look, I contemplated coloring her hair as well. When she was 28 I decided that it was finally time for the bottle. I told Lindsay about my plan and she nodded yes to the proposition of change. After all, Lindsay was entitled to maintain her youthful glow!

I spoke to our hairstylist, Kevin, and he recommended a rinse for Miss Lindsay's hair. He has affectionately called her this name since she was a little girl. (We have followed him throughout his career to several salons and Lindsay looks forward to her haircuts and seeing Kevin.) Kevin is a true artist. While talking to Lindsay as she sits in the chair, or wiggles from side to side, the result is always a masterpiece. Kevin is like Edward Scissorhands; beauty is created every time. Lindsay enjoys the compliments on her fresh haircut and style from the other professionals in the salon as well. So, of course, Kevin's advice concerning the hair rinse was taken under advisement. With a bit of trepidation, I became a colorist and my first client was Lindsay.

This new project began in the master bathroom where Lindsay sat on the step leading to the bathtub. I gave her an old t-shirt of mine to wear and then gloved up and proceeded with the experiment. Lindsay sat quite still and allowed me to proceed. I was careful not to get the dark color on her skin and kept telling her that it was "beautification time." Except for scratching her head a few times and getting black goo all over her hand, she was actually very cooperative. The rinse stayed on for about ten minutes and then we proceeded to the shower. Lindsay did her usual routine of holding onto the handle of the door and placing the other hand on the grab bar. However, as I prepared to wash off the mixture, Lindsay leaned backward and transferred the mess onto me. The showerhead came to the rescue as I rinsed myself in addition to Lindsay's hair. While engaged in this process there was much splashing of the color all over me, the walls and, of course, Lindsay. We were quite the sight. But it's really worth it since the color typically stays on for about three weeks before those pesky grays start to rear their ugly heads once again.

In addition to showering, shaving is also a part of Lindsay's hygiene. This can prove to be an adventure, too. Showering is a two-for-one deal. I find that I, too, can shower at the same time as Lindsay, making the procedure time efficient. After all the washing and shampooing and conditioning are completed, the real test is shaving her legs and underarms. It's a good thing she is quite secure with her balance since I have to move around to be sure that her legs are completely smooth. After this, I then remove any unwanted hair from her arms and face. Since excessive hair growth is a component of MSS, Lindsay's entire body has way too much of it. Shaving is basically a maintenance procedure, due to the fact that Lindsay has been undergoing laser hair removal from these areas for several years. The procedure is quite painless and Lindsay is extremely cooperative. Laser hair removal should permanently resolve this issue, but, unfortunately, it doesn't. (Due to MSS, I suppose that permanent removal is not a reality.) However, the laser has definitely slowed the process and actually removed and thinned the hair from her face and arms.

"Yet again, as the arthritis grew more severe, the bike riding diminished."

Even though I am acutely aware of the many life experiences that Lindsay will never partake in, I am also grateful for the things that she has accomplished. When Lindsay was six years old she participated in an ice skating program at Farr Conservatory. This organization provided many activities for children with disabilities. Lindsay used her walker to move about on the ice, and yes, she actually wore ice skates. She could only maneuver a few steps, but it was a sight to behold. She enjoyed the program for several years. Then Lindsay moved on to "Horseback Riding for Handicappers" at the Bloomfield Open Hunt Club. Lindsay rode a horse for one hour a week while three volunteers walked next to the horse to ensure her safety. The volunteers were incredible people, and without their assistance Lindsay would never have been able to ride. They led her around the barn area and talked to her as she rode. She enjoyed these weekly experiences for ten years, until arthritic hips prevented further riding. Another one bites the dust.

Riding an adaptive bicycle was also a great activity for Lindsay. Her feet were strapped onto elongated pedals that had Velcro straps on each side. A pulley system helped move the pedals smoothly, initiating momentum. Lindsay wore a seat belt around her waist and held onto the handlebars by herself. She needed only a little assistance to propel herself forward and then she was off, sailing smoothly down the street. It was a joy to walk next to her and talk as we navigated around the neighborhood. Yet again, as the arthritis grew more severe, the bike riding diminished. Even after Lindsay started to receive a regimen of cortisone injections and felt a great deal of relief, she still could not ride the bicycle again. The rise and fall of the pedaling action proved to be too difficult. The pain crept in and the bike was out.

In order to continue the joy she felt while riding I did the next best thing. I had often seen people riding bikes with their children in tow on a variety of adaptive carriages. So I bought a Cannondale carrier that attached to my bicycle seat and soon Lindsay was rolling once again. She used a seat belt to keep her inside the carrier, and she enjoyed the view of the entire neighborhood. It was great. What made it even better was that Todd, Chad, or Eli could easily take Lindsay for a ride as well. Their rides, however, were not as calm and serene as mine. They would ride like madmen, zig-zagging the carrier and making Lindsay laugh. The more wild the ride, the more hysterical Lindsay would become. She was absolutely elated to be driven around by her crazy brothers.

To this day they still take her for rides, although they have progressed to jet skis. At first the idea of her going out on the water with the boys was quite frightening. However, Jeffrey and I have by now become accustomed to this ritual. Most summer vacations we rent a house up north on a lake where rental jet skis are available. Of course, the boys ride around the lake with great enthusiasm. They hold onto Lindsay and cruise slowly while Lindsay makes sounds that we have never heard before. These are sounds of utter happiness and it makes us happy as well.

When not in the water, the boys like to push Lindsay's wheelchair around in a variety of directions and speeds in order to elicit laughter. We all enjoy hearing Lindsay's deep belly laughs. We can be walking in a mall, on the sidewalk, or in a parking lot and they will suddenly start zig-zagging the chair or propelling it forward so that Lindsay gets a rise from the acceleration. Lindsay's favorite wheelchair activity takes place on an incline, like the driveway. Jeffrey or one of the boys will spin the chair around, allowing Lindsay to careen down the slope until they catch her. Of course, her laughter is infectious and everyone knows that these wild moments are heartwarming and scary at the same time.

Chapter Twelve

"I would tell Dr. Gilmore repeatedly that there were no coincidences in life, only plans set into motion on a grand scale by God."

After Benn Gilmore saved Lindsay's life, there was built-in loyalty forever. It didn't matter where he moved his practice, we were sure to follow. Lindsay and I were groupies of his Ear, Nose, and Throat practice and there was no return from this infatuation. Benn definitely cast a spell, not only on our family, but on so many others as well. This knowledgeable man attracted patients from near and far. Sitting in his waiting room, people would talk about the distances they drove just to have their children or themselves examined by Dr. Gilmore. And they were willing to wait, since they knew he would give them his undivided attention. I never felt rushed or short changed for time when Benn was examining Lindsay or one of the boys. Benn had created a true following because all of his patients knew that he had a special touch.

After Lindsay's long hospitalization and subsequent recovery, I reminded Benn several times that I truly believed his move from California to Detroit, at that specific time, was divine intervention. Benn knew Lindsay's medical condition and he was alarmed by the mistreatment she had received at the hands of the so-called professionals at Henry Ford Hospital. However, he believed it was merely a coincidence that he arrived on the scene just in the nick of time to help Lindsay. I would tell him repeatedly that there were no coincidences in life, only plans set into motion on a grand scale by God. He would simply smile and give me a little laugh. Benn was an atheist. Most of his patients were not. We were all aware of his innate wisdom and felt that he was truly blessed.

Only many years later did Benn come to the realization that, indeed, there was a God, and he was here to do His work. Benn had always been a consummate professional and he even went abroad to teach other doctors, bringing medical supplies to needy areas. Then he and his wife, Kathleen, organized Christian missionary trips to serve a larger group in many different countries. Benn became a regular at church and even began to teach Sunday school on a weekly basis.

He now studies both the New and the Old Testament and also gleans knowledge from rabbis in addition to priests and pastors. His thirst for understanding and harmony in this world is quite apparent. Benn invariably understands his patients' perspectives when it comes to faith. He once told me that when he found religion he discussed this awakening with one of his patients. She commented that it was no surprise to her; she had been praying all along for Benn and had been looking forward to the day when it finally arrived.

Another day arrived for Benn, a sadder one for his patients, a day I'd long anticipated with fear and trepidation: the day he announced his retirement. Lindsay had done so well throughout the years and the thought of forging a new relationship with a virtual stranger was a bit daunting. After all, Benn was the one who had performed several successful surgeries on Lindsay. Even when she needed eye surgery he was there to intubate Lindsay to ensure that her airway was not damaged. Who could take his place? Would I be able to trust this individual? How was I going to make Lindsay understand that Benn was off to new adventures, intending to help people in a different capacity? Benn had recently taken on a new partner, Esmael Amjad, and we had met him only briefly in the hallway. He seemed very nice and cordial, but he was basically a stranger. I did know this much; if Benn brought him into his practice, then he certainly had to be upstanding.

An invitation arrived at the beginning of December announcing both Benn's and his partner, Dr. Lacivita's, retirement. They were hosting an open house for one last hurrah with all of their patients. Unfortunately, we were not able to attend. Our family was headed to Israel to visit Todd and his wife, Chana Tova. We were leaving at the exact time the reception was beginning. Marty Levinson and his son, Josh, attended and reported that it was an incredible event with over 600 people in attendance who wanted to say goodbye and thank you to Benn. There were smiles, good wishes, and lots of tears.

Jeffrey and I wanted to do something special for Benn and so, upon our return, we invited him and Kathleen out to dinner. As we were catching up, I told Benn that I had recently taken Lindsay to Dr. Amjad for a checkup. While driving to the appointment I kept reminding Lindsay that Benn would not be there to greet her; instead, a new doctor would be helping her from now on. She appeared to comprehend my words and I didn't notice anything unusual about her behavior while waiting to be seen. The staff greeted Lindsay with smiles and pleasant conversation, as usual. When Lindsay's name was called, we walked slowly to the examination room. Minutes later, Dr. Amjad appeared at the door and the introductions began. Then, when he approached Lindsay to say hello, she turned to me and began to cry. This was completely out of character, and we realized then that Lindsay was acutely aware of Benn's absence.

After a few moments she regained her composure and so did Dr. Amjad. It was obvious this scenario had been played out with other patients. I could see the gentle side of this new physician who was going to watch over Lindsay's health. He was a soft spoken man who displayed compassion and interest for his patients. Lindsay felt his warmth and, at the end of the appointment, she waved goodbye. She never shed a tear again in his office.

As I discussed this scenario with Benn he did not say a word. He hung his head and tears welled up in his eyes. I suspect Benn's retirement has been bittersweet.

"He listened intently as I conveyed the issues related to MSS and asked if he could help make it possible for Lindsay to walk."

When Lindsay was quite young I received a phone call from Brent Cooper, a high school friend who happened to be attending chiropractic school. He told me about a local chiropractor whose technique might be beneficial to Lindsay's well-being. The name of this man was Dr. George Goodheart. His practice was on Mack Avenue in Grosse Pointe. I did not know a thing about chiropractic medicine, so Brent told me to read a book by Edgar Casey that discussed the benefits of spinal alignment to the overall health of the individual. There was information about osteopathic medicine and the training one receives in chiropractic school.

Many concepts started to make sense. However, I was still quite apprehensive. It took several months before I picked up the phone to make an appointment. Much to my surprise, I was told that Dr. Goodheart was not taking on any new patients since he was only working part-time. I called Brent back and told him the news. We decided that I should try one more time—the difference being that this time I would tell the receptionist about Lindsay's condition. Since Marshall-Smith Syndrome was so rare, we thought it might just be the catalyst to get an appointment. On this second call, the receptionist said she would apprise the doctor of Lindsay's unique condition and then get back to me. I had never used the MSS card before then, but now it seemed appropriate. A few days later, I received the green light. Dr. Goodheart said that he would be interested in treating Lindsay.

The office was lined with patients awaiting their appointments. After an hour, we were escorted into an examination room and I was handed a gown for Lindsay to wear. Thus wardrobed, I propped her up on the table.

Dr. Goodheart had striking dark hair and a tan to compliment it. He listened intently as I conveyed the issues related to MSS and asked if he could make it possible for Lindsay to walk. By this point, she had been going to physical therapy for several years and was still not able to walk without assistance. I wasn't sure if she would ever reach this milestone, but I was not about to give up either. Dr. Goodheart stated that there were multiple approaches to the problem and set out to explain cranial sacral therapy as well as Applied Kinesiology. (I later discovered that his books and approach were taught in many chiropractic schools.)

With cranial sacral therapy, apparently the sutures of the head can be moved in order to relieve pressure on other parts of the body. There are those in the medical community that believe these sutures do not move after infancy. According to his friend, Dr. Donald McDowall, however:

> In 1964 he began a series of revolutionary observations about muscle function and health, which he introduced to the world as Applied Kinesiology (AK). It all began with a research manual, the first of over 30 he would write. Progressive chiropractic physicians around the country quickly recognized the groundbreaking nature of his work in the care and healing of their patients. This group, who called themselves "The Dirty Dozen," established what is now the International College of Applied Kinesiology, which has grown to more than 600 members in the U.S. and over 3,000 worldwide. Every day millions of people worldwide receive the benefit of Dr. Goodheart's work.

And, thankfully, Lindsay was one of these lucky people.

Many different machines lined the room. A computer assessed Lindsay's spinal alignment, or lack thereof. He had Lindsay stand up straight and then proceeded to run a wand down her spine to gain valuable measurements. The computer then let him know which specific vertebrae were out of whack. All of these things might help Lindsay to walk, but it would take some time before we saw results. When Dr. Goodheart spoke about his various techniques I was mesmerized. I didn't have a clue these types of treatments even existed. It was all foreign to me, but I made sure that with each consecutive visit Dr. Goodheart broke down the precise components of his technique. I wanted to be sure to ask the right questions and he was more than willing to answer them.

During the ensuing years, I became familiar with the meridians of the body. I frequently consulted his chart to find out how they played into one's overall health. I also learned that when a person is exhibiting pain in a specific area, such as a leg, that it's not uncommon to discover the cause of this problem in another area of the body. An individual with leg pain might find relief when his neck is manipulated in a specific manner, for example. In the end, relief may be found rather quickly with a cursory examination of the entire body. Dr. Goodheart was an extremely interesting man and Lindsay and I listened intently to each word as he worked expertly to give her more mobility. Lindsay saw Dr. Goodheart faithfully for twenty years, usually once a month. He was delighted to see her progress and even more elated to hear her voice. It's interesting that her most clearly spoken word is "good." It makes me wonder. And this man definitely had a true and good heart. He was inspired by his father, who was also a chiropractor. Dr. Goodheart dedicated his career to helping individuals alleviate pain and correct troublesome conditions.

Toward the end of his "semi-retired" status, I noticed that he was slowing down and had a shuffle instead of exhibiting a precise gait when he walked. It made me very sad. He was in his 80s and was still determined to help patients. I was quite familiar with "the shuffle" because my father and father-in-law both acquired this pattern of walking as they aged. It signaled the slow descent to more severe problems. Eventually, Dr. Goodheart could no longer maneuver Lindsay on the table and I helped in this area. One day after I arrived home from teaching, Jeffrey told me that he'd received a phone call from Dr. Goodheart's office. His receptionist said that the good doctor was not going to have office hours anymore. What an interesting way to say that he was in ill health. Dr. Goodheart died on March 5, 2008. He was 89 years young.

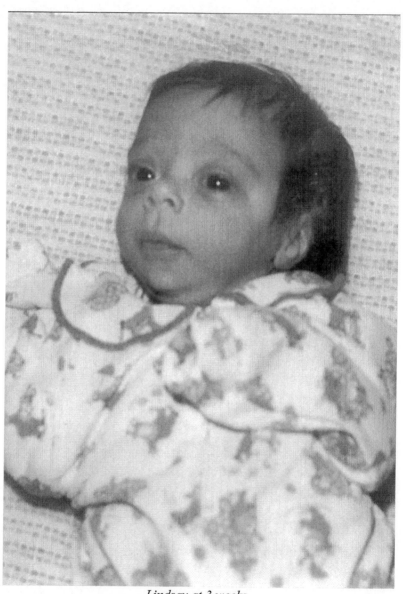

Lindsay at 3 weeks.

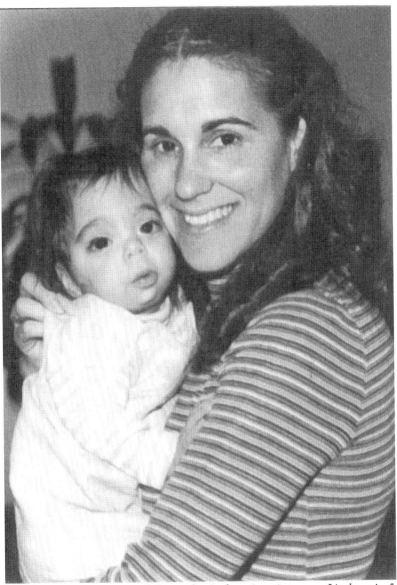

Lindsay and Judi—one of the author's favorite pictures. Lindsay is 5 months old.

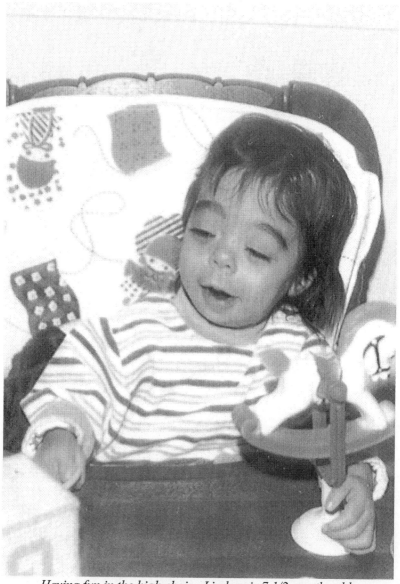

Having fun in the high chair. Lindsay is 7 1/2 months old.

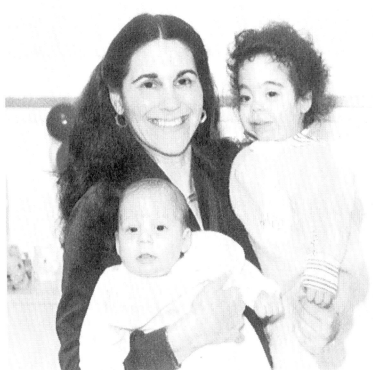

Lindsay at 16 months. She likes her new brother Todd.

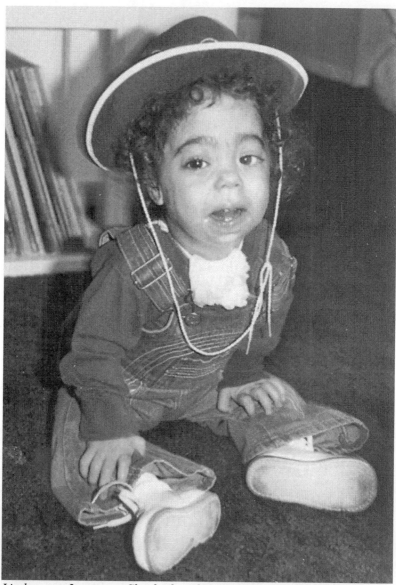

Lindsay at 2 years. She had a damp gauze covering her trach (it provides moisture).

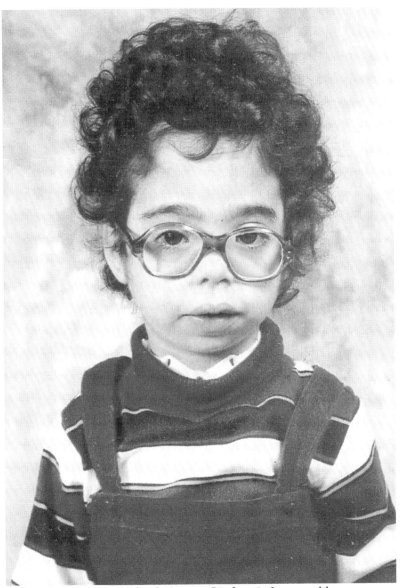

A serious school picture. Lindsay is 3 years old.

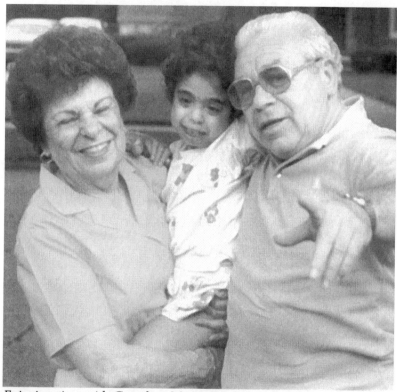

Enjoying time with Grandma Marian and Grandpa Bob. Lindsay is 5 years old.

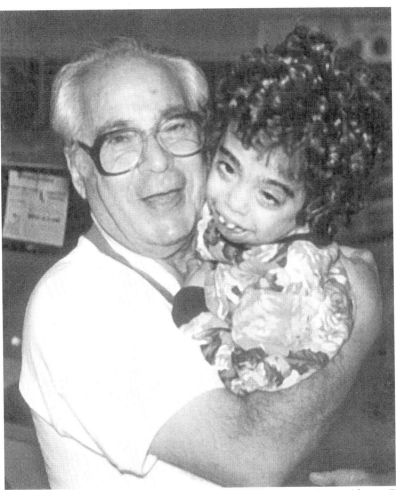

Grandpa Sam having fun at the bowling alley with Lindsay. She is 7 years old.

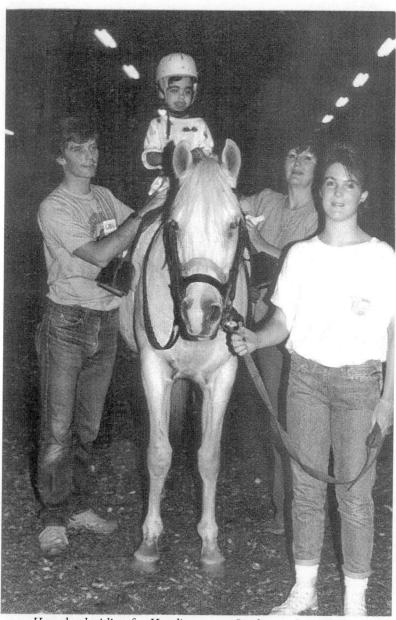

Horseback riding for Handicappers. Lindsay is 8 years old.

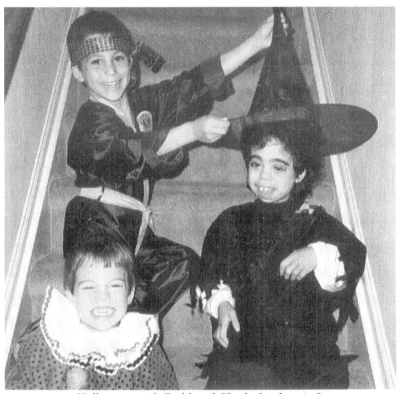

Halloween with Todd and Chad. Lindsay is 8.

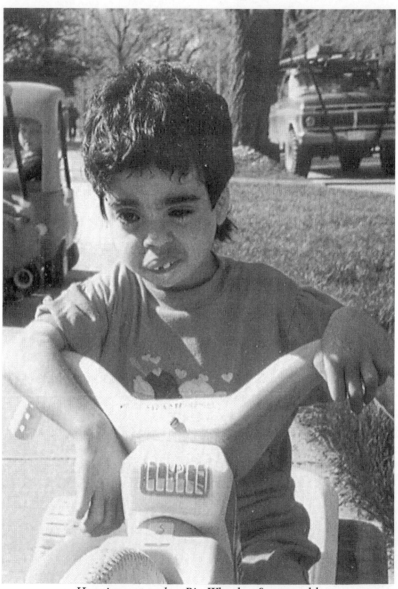

Hanging out on her Big Wheel at 9 years old.

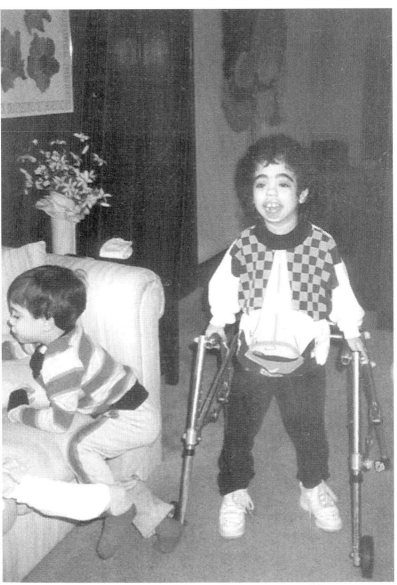

Cruising along with her walker - 10 years old.

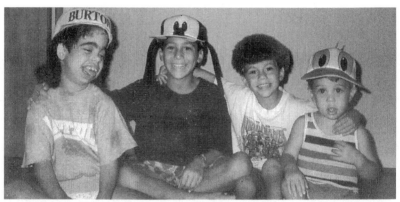

Having fun with Todd, Chad and Eli - Lindsay is 11 years old.

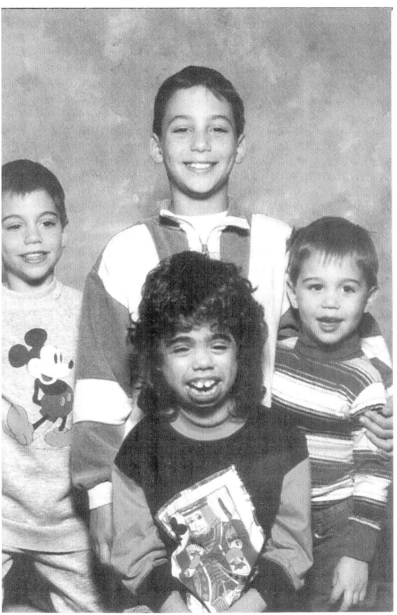

Smiles all around with "The Crew." Lindsay is 12.

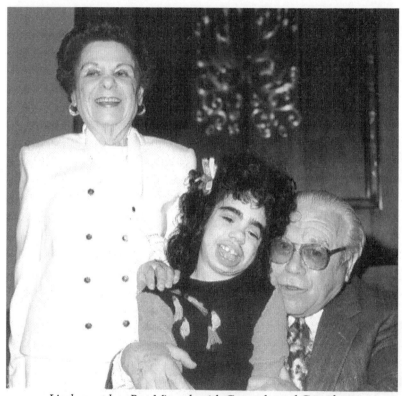

Lindsay at her Bat Mitzvah with Granpda and Grandma.

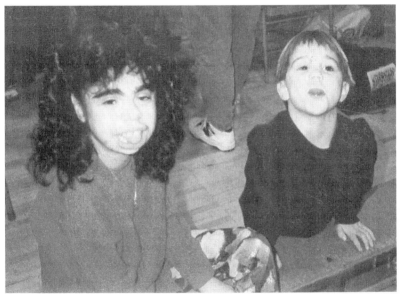

Sharing the bleachers with Eli at Todd's basketball game. Lindsay is 14 years old.

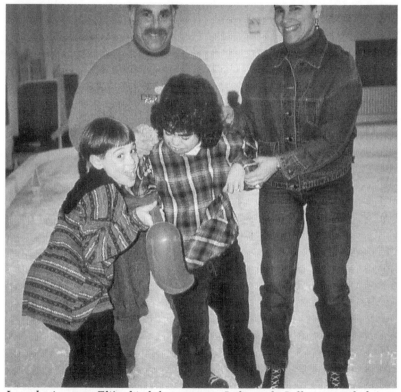

Ice skating at Eli's birthday party. Judi and Jeffrey are helping. Lindsay is 16.

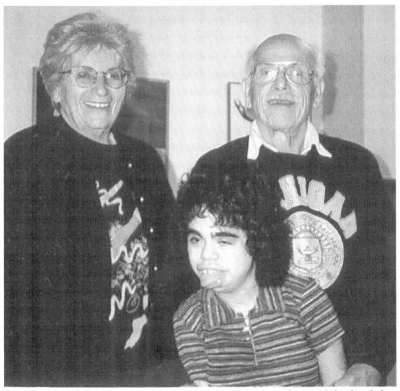

Lou and Claire having fun with Lindsay at her 18th birthday celebration.

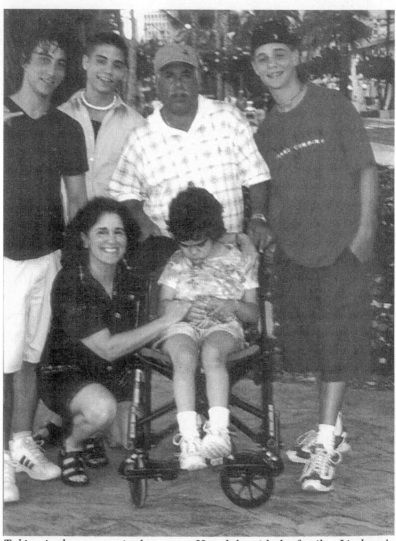

Taking in the scenery in downtown Honolulu with the family. Lindsay is being camera shy - 21 years.

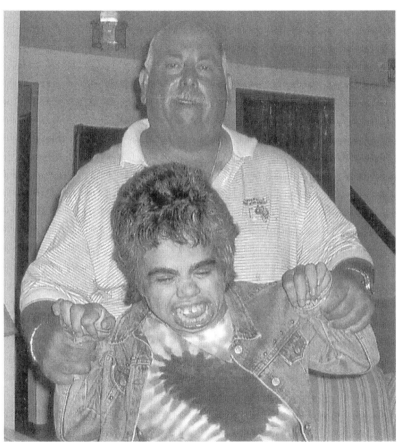

Having a good laugh, walking with Jeffrey around the house we rented on Burt Lake, Cheboygan, Michigan. Lindsay is 22.

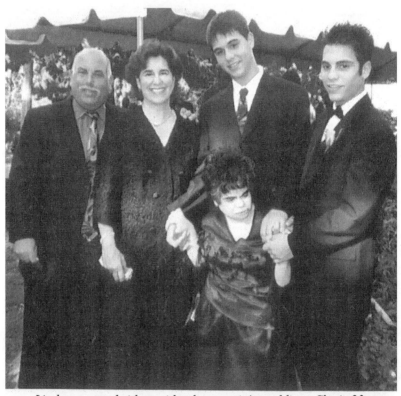

Lindsay was a bridesmaid at her cousin's wedding. She is 23.

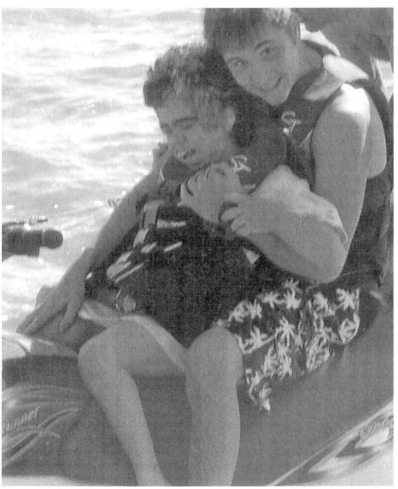

Eli and Lindsay getting ready to Jet-Ski. Lindsay is 25.

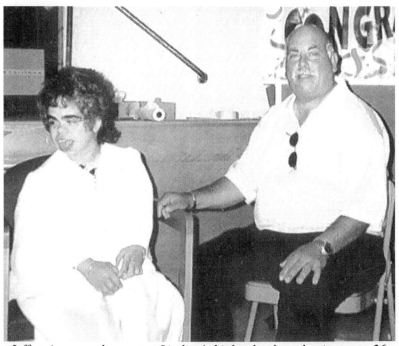

Jeffrey is a proud parent at Lindsay's high school graduation - age 26.

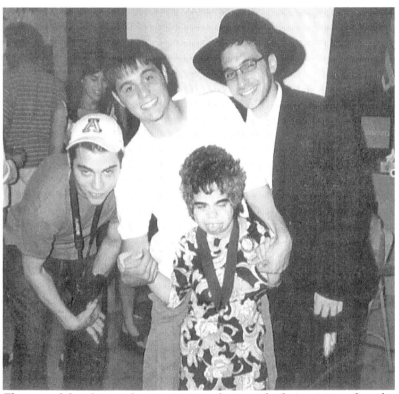

The proud brothers take a winning photo with their sister after the graduation ceremony.

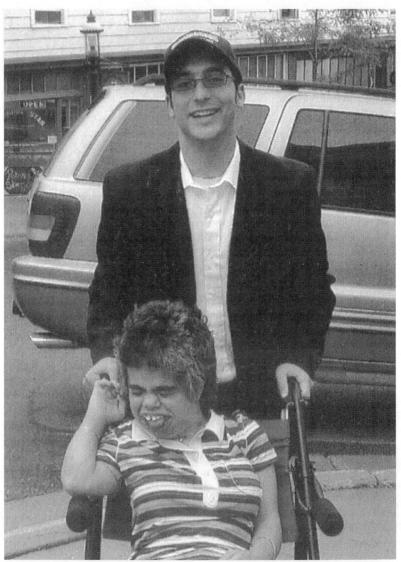

Strolling the streets of Petoskey, Michigan with Todd. Lindsay is 26.

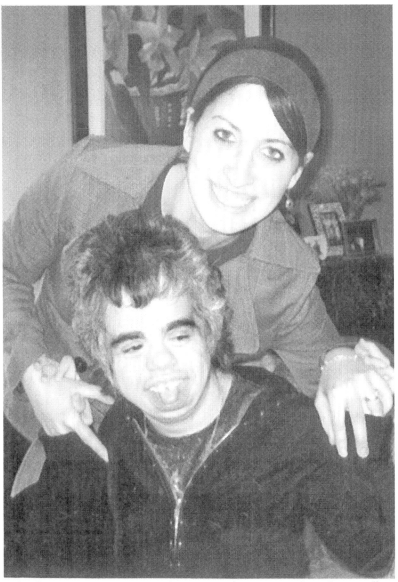

Lindsay, age 27, is taking Chana Tova, her sister in-law, for a walk.

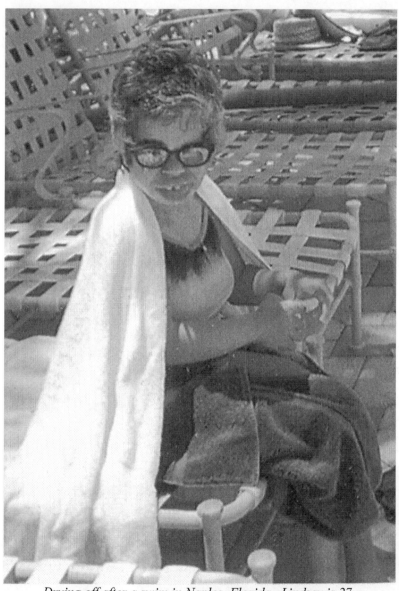

Drying off after a swim in Naples, Florida. Lindsay is 27.

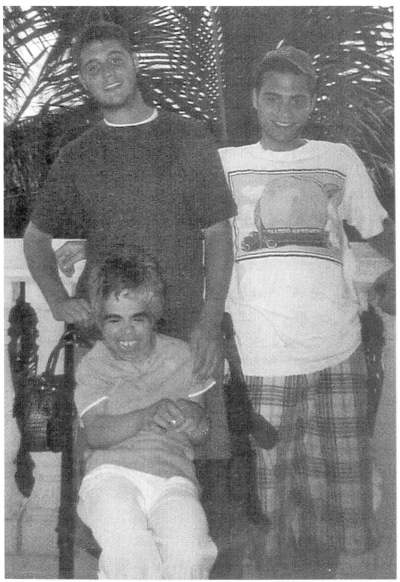

Getting ready for a night on the town with Eli and Chad in Naples, Florida.

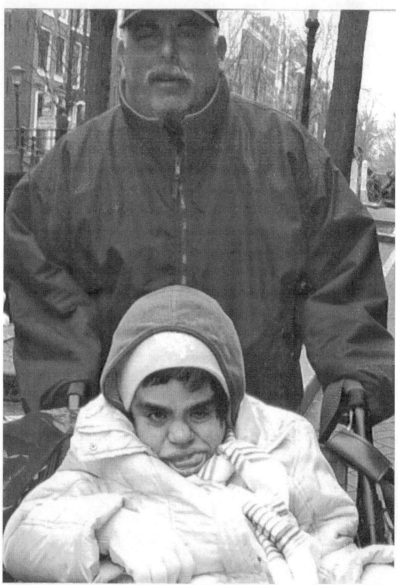

Lindsay, age 28, and Jeffrey walking along a canal in Amsterdam.

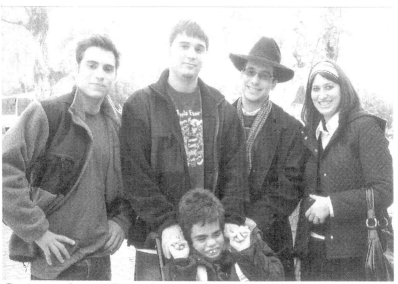

Getting ready to walk into the Jerusalem Zoo (Todd, Chana Tova, Chad and Eli). Lindsay is 28.

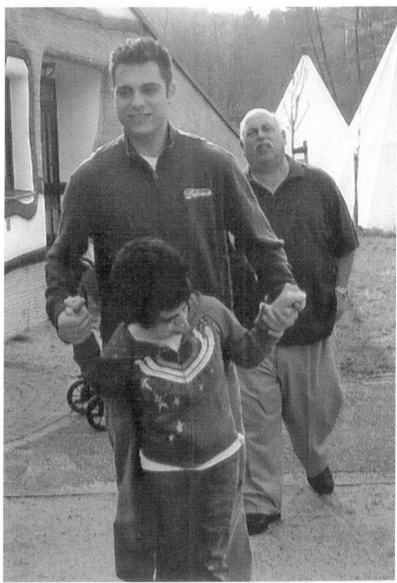

Lindsay, 29, Chad and Jeffrey walking around the grounds of Kindervallei in Valkenburg, Netherlands.

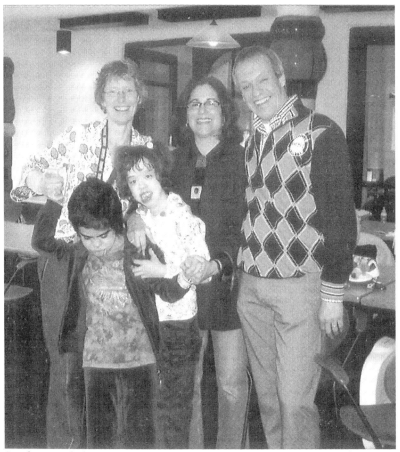

Lindsay with her new friend Nina at the Kindervallei in Valkenburg. Judi, Sonja and Karel (Nina's parents).

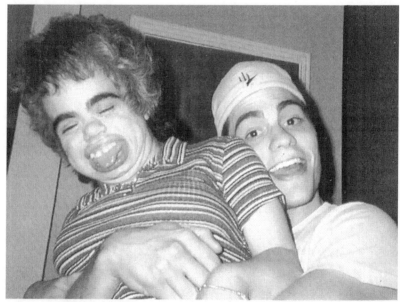

Lindsay, 30, enjoying a "special lift" from Chad.

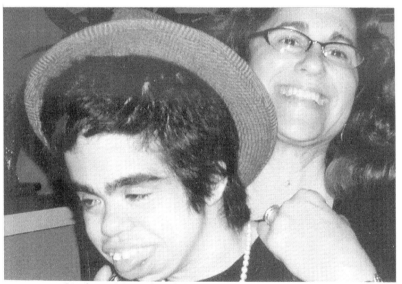

Lindsay, 31, and Judi having fun at a family party.

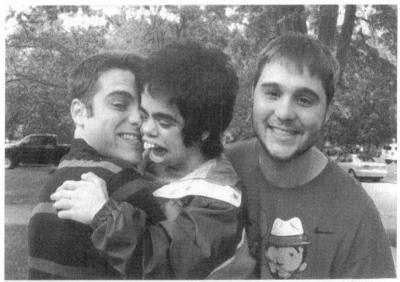

Chad, Eli and Lindsay, 32, enjoying themselves in front of our house.

Chapter Thirteen

"Not only do we need to feel secure, but we also need to know that Lindsay likes the person."

It has always been a difficult task finding reliable people to watch Lindsay when Jeffrey and I want to go out for an evening. Our pool of resources is quite limited. Not only do we need to feel secure, but we also need to know that Lindsay likes the person. Her end of the deal is easy—she sizes up a candidate right away. If she likes someone she will begin to smile and even extend a hand toward them. However, if she doesn't like a potential companion, she will give us a verbal signal by complaining. It's really quite that simple. Lindsay has built-in radar for people and she senses their feelings toward her in a short amount of time. After wonderful experiences with several neighbors we were in a bind to match their expertise. Kelly Schrubba and Mandy Friedenberg were expert caregivers and mature as well. They watched all four kids and made it look easy. But when they left school and began their careers, our time was done. So the hunt began with her school programs. Who could be more qualified than the aides working with Lindsay on a daily basis?

Lindsay's first "official" school experience was at Avery Elementary in Oak Park. Since she had been identified as POHI (Physically and Otherwise Health Impaired), Avery seemed the best choice. However, they did not feel comfortable with her trach and did not want any of the responsibility for making sure it was properly suctioned.

In order for her to attend the program, I agreed to stay in the hall while she spent half a day in school. I assured them I would be ready if any suctioning was required. I could tell that most of the staff was ill at ease with Lindsay from the start. That, along with the fact that Lindsay had to adjust to a new situation and new people, naturally put me on guard. It was obvious that I would not find any caregivers in this school.

My perceptions were not wrong. Several months into the school year I was notified that they felt Lindsay was not appropriate for their program and should probably attend Einstein Center for more severely impaired individuals. They said the program at Einstein was better equipped to handle fragile medical conditions and that Lindsay was not responding in the manner anticipated. My mind was spinning. All I could think was, "Lindsay is three years old and already she's being demoted."

I immediately went to the pay phone in the hallway to contact the Director of Special Education for the Berkley School District, which includes Avery. He more or less repeated the same spiel; however, I was in no mood to accept their decision. Lindsay was very young and making progress, but they had already determined that she did not have the cognitive capability to function in their program? No way. I kept reiterating that she needed a chance, and several months was not long enough to properly evaluate her potential. After promoting Lindsay like I was a cheerleader on the sidelines, I hung up the phone. I was completely rattled. I needed time to think.

I didn't want Lindsay to stay in a program where she wasn't wanted but, on the other hand, I didn't think she belonged in a center program. There was no middle ground. I decided to visit Einstein. Once there, I believed with all my heart that Lindsay didn't fit in with the population. This program served the needs of severely impaired individuals. I wanted Lindsay to maximize her potential and be with people who were making considerable strides and people who were good role models. Still, after much contemplation, and few options, I reluctantly enrolled her at Einstein.

The program was headed by Dr. Barry Berlin. He had innovative ideas that incorporated peers from the elementary school working closely with the students who were challenged. Lindsay began the program in 1982. This was not the norm for most center-based facilities catering to severely multiply impaired students. The program had community-based outings, a kitchen where cooking skills were taught, plus occupational and physical therapy. Barry kept the morale upbeat at all times. He was an involved administrator and knew each of his students personally. In this program Lindsay met Juan Strayham and Emma Hawthorne. They had been working as classroom aides and she saw them every day. They forged a solid relationship, enjoying each other's company and Juan started to watch Lindsay at home while she still had her trach. He wasn't intimidated by this responsibility and learned quickly. It was obvious that he truly loved Lindsay and he treated her as if she was his own daughter.

When Lindsay began the program, I sat outside of her classroom for several weeks until I was assured that everyone felt comfortable with her care. I also had to come to terms with the fact that I would be leaving Lindsay there every day. The staff was very conscientious and loving. For a first time experience this was a model. Lindsay's teachers, Lori Miller and Ruth Hurvitz, were truly exceptional with their students. I realized I had completely misjudged the program during that first visit.

After several months, however, it became clear to the school psychologist, Fran King, that Lindsay was functioning on a higher level than most of her counterparts and actually belonged at Avery School. This was great news to hear and we decided to fight the system from within. Fran periodically tested Lindsay and stated that consistent patterns were observed and, if they continued, she would file the necessary paperwork for Lindsay's transfer back to Avery. The staff believed it was Lindsay's right to be in a program that best suited her needs, and they were more than happy to assist in this battle.

After a year at Einstein Center, as part of this wonderfully supportive program, Lindsay was welcomed back at Avery. Juan transitioned Lindsay to the school and made sure she felt comfortable. Lindsay didn't have her trach anymore, so their concerns about keeping her airway suctioned were now gone. She was placed with a new teacher. Marsha Snyder was absolutely great with Lindsay. She was warm-hearted and nurturing. Marsha's classroom was stimulating and the students made progress in her charge. The therapists, Robin Cutler and Mary Pat Reichel, were highly skilled and Lindsay was happy in this environment. It was as if the past problems had never existed.

Lindsay enjoyed her time at Avery with her buddy, Josh. They rode the bus together. Her years at Avery turned out to be quite pleasant. When this program ended, however, Lindsay embarked on a new journey once again.

There was no hesitation this time when it was recommended that Lindsay should attend a center program at Roosevelt Middle School, and Emma was there as well. Emma had the reputation of taking a hard line. She was demanding of her students, and I was a bit apprehensive when she began to work with Lindsay. But I quickly learned that she was a softie under that stern veneer. Emma was deeply loved by Lindsay and the feeling was mutual. Emma challenged Lindsay to do her best. They would shop, go to restaurants, visit Emma's family, and she even had Lindsay sleep over so that Jeffrey and I could do a bit of traveling. We knew Lindsay was safe and having a good time. The two of them shared a rich slice of life until Emma became ill. She battled cancer several times but, ultimately, its grip proved too strong. Emma passed away and, sadly, another close relationship ended for Lindsay.

Willie Turner, our housekeeper, was also quite attached to Lindsay. For many years she watched Lindsay and the boys whenever she was available. The kids loved her southern style of cooking and couldn't wait to eat her fried chicken and creamed corn. Willie would walk with Lindsay on top of her feet, holding her hands at the same time. This absolutely made her crack up. Each of the boys took turns as well. Time marched forward, however, and Willie finally had to retire due to health issues.

At this point, I contacted JARC (Jewish Association for Residential Care) about finding a caregiver for Lindsay. JARC is responsible for the interviewing and screening of these individuals. However, it's not an easy task to match a client with an employee. After waiting for nearly a year, we finally received a phone call. We were told that a young lady by the name of Katie Cooper would be a perfect fit.

Katie was 21 years old when she befriended Lindsay and, indeed, it was a great match. Lindsay immediately gravitated toward Katie and they shared many good times together. Katie was mature for her age and didn't have a problem taking Lindsay to the bathroom, as well as addressing all of her feminine needs. She was a breath of fresh air and we were so grateful to have her in Lindsay's life. Katie attended Wayne State University and was in her senior year. She was in the process of applying to graduate school in the Speech and Language Pathology program. Lindsay and Katie had a true connection. Katie was irresistible; she was energetic, warm, and friendly. They ran around town and had a blast together. She would take Lindsay to her mother's house and to visit her friends. She also had Lindsay over to her house to hang out with her dogs. Jeffrey and I implicitly trusted Katie and, she too, cared for Lindsay when we went out of town. In a pinch, Katie could also keep an eye on Eli, too.

After graduate school, however, the writing was on the wall once again. We knew Katie would be entering the workforce and that she would be helping many students along the way. It was her turn in the world and, eventually, she was no longer able to watch Lindsay for us. And so, after a three year relationship, we sadly said goodbye. Katie still keeps in touch with us, always asking about Lindsay's well-being.

Throughout the years, there have been many "companions" who have touched Lindsay's life. Most of them are wonderful people but, for a variety of reasons, couldn't continue this line of work. That's definitely one of the most frustrating and saddest things for Lindsay,

Jeffrey, and me. Relationships don't last and, as fast as people enter her life, they are gone.

One constant in her life has been her school programs, the teachers, and aides. I have never seen more dedicated people in my life. To think that they chose to work with this population is unbelievable. It's not an easy task and they have to deal with ten to twelve students every day. When Lindsay started Einstein Center, Ruth Hurwitz was her teacher. I remember when she asked me what I wanted my daughter to achieve. My reply was the usual—I wanted Lindsay to be healthy and happy. But I added that if she could learn to walk and hold my hand that would be nice, too. And, even for a stretch, I hoped to hear Lindsay say, "Mom." I don't think I was asking for too much. Lindsay certainly was able to achieve two of those goals and she always seemed to know that it made me very happy. As for the third ... I have never heard that word. My consolation is that Lindsay definitely understands that's my role.

Upon entering Roosevelt Middle School, Sandy Stehlin became Lindsay's teacher. She was a vibrant and active woman. There were trips to the zoo and the beach, and Sandy also involved her students in scouting. In fact, the class went for an overnight in Metamora, about 25 miles north, for their annual scouting excursion. There was horseback riding, a bonfire, and communing with nature. Sandy kept pushing her students to communicate and to learn as much as possible. It was obvious that she, too, loved her job. There were even "grandma and grandpa" volunteers in the classroom. The really nice thing about the program was that Emma and Juan were there for several years. Emma then followed Lindsay to high school when she was transferred.

Mike Bliss was in charge of the high school program and he had a gentle approach with his students. The classroom was always bustling with activity. While attending Oak Park High School, Lindsay definitely learned a lot about cooking. The aides would help her measure ingredients, pour the contents of a recipe into a bowl or pot, stir, and then watch over the final product. There was a lot of hand-over-hand assistance, but Lindsay enjoyed the thrill of these cooking adventures. Any time I had to pick Lindsay up early, I always smelled wonderful aromas as I walked down the hallway of the school. Unfortunately, the center was slated to close at the end of Lindsay's first year and this sent everyone into an uproar.

> *"I always felt a tug at my heartstrings whenever Lindsay had to make a transition to a new setting. Change is difficult for many people; however, when dealing with impairments, this compounds the situation."*

All of the students had to be placed into new programs. The staff, too, was in a bind as every one of them had to seek new employment. Lindsay and Robbie, a long time friend and fellow student, began attending Wing Lake. The other students headed to a variety of other programs around the county. Robbie's mother, Carol, and I went to observe the Wing Lake program before making our final decision. Right from the start we were impressed with Ray Hooten's classroom. It was a nice departure to have another male teacher, and he certainly played an active role with his students. He was a compassionate and dedicated teacher. Ray's classroom was well organized and learning was at the forefront each day.

I always felt a tug at my heartstrings whenever Lindsay had to make a transition to a new setting. Change is difficult for many people; however, when dealing with impairments, this compounds the situation. Lindsay takes a while to adjust to new people and different routines. She keenly observes her surroundings and needs to put everything into perspective. Fortunately, Emma helped with the transition. She rode with Lindsay on the bus to Andover High School, a public school in Bloomfield Hills. Several days a week they would sit in Ray's class and take in the change of scenery. Ray also had an aide in his classroom, Willie. He was a great asset to this program since he was quite attuned to each of the students. Willie was like a cuddly bear: tough on the outside and gentle as a lamb on the inside. He knew how to handle difficult situations with a calm demeanor. Anyone who works with special needs students has to be special themselves. If not, they don't belong in the field. Patience and perseverance are key to a successful classroom atmosphere. And Ray's class fit nicely into this mold. Shortly, however, Ray was asked to return to the main facility at Wing Lake to teach a different class. Since Lindsay's program was a satellite of Wing Lake, another teacher from the district was going to replace Ray. Once again, I became quite nervous for Lindsay. More changes and adjustments were in line.

Kathie Schuld came on the scene with zest and vigor. She had many years of experience and wanted the students to make substantial gains. Kathie transitioned into Ray's room smoothly and made sure that the students were secure in their routines. Naturally, she conferenced with Ray to be certain that the students were progressing appropriately. Every teacher brings a wealth of background experience into their respective domain. After a short while, Kathie began to introduce her own unique style to the class and the students adapted quickly.

With the availability of technology there were always plenty of pictures to document most of the classroom activities. I could see that Lindsay was immersed in the tasks that became the focus of each lesson. Birthdays were also a big deal at Wing Lake. Since I loved these special times as well, cakes, cookies, or brownies were brought in for the class, and there was always a photo album sent home with a narrative describing the festivities. Food preparation was also a mainstay and everyone delighted in the treats that resulted from this exercise.. Adaptive switches were used for blenders, mixers and most kitchen appliances, so the students could partake in the activity.

Additionally, Kathie promoted peer assistance in the classroom and many of the regular education students rotated in and out of her room. Everyone benefited from this routine. The general education students commented that they learned a great deal from each of the students they worked with, and Kathie's students enjoyed a refreshing change of pace with their peers. I always felt that Lindsay was making nice progress in Kathie's room.

She was so proud of her students; her dedication was evident.

Then, on June 5th 2005, after eight years at Wing Lake, Lindsay graduated. What an amazing day! Our entire family attended and Todd even flew in from Israel. Friends came as well and there was a great deal of excitement in the air. The cafeteria was decorated with banners and flowers. There were only three graduates, each dressed in a cap and gown. (Of course, I had to hunt down a small one and have it shortened so that Lindsay could walk unimpeded during the processional.) We were so very proud of her and could not believe that it was her turn to wear the graduate's uniform.

The significance of the moment was not lost on a single person that day as speeches were delivered and diplomas were handed out to each of the three graduates. That was the moment the flood gates opened with a vengeance for me. I realized it was a celebration, but leaving such a solid institution was very sad and quite scary. Wing Lake had served as Lindsay's extended family and now it was all coming to an end. The tears flowed both for the things that Lindsay had accomplished and for the things that would never be. During the festivities, Lindsay's smile was bright and contagious, as usual. I don't know if she fully comprehended that her program at Wing Lake would be ending shortly, but I already felt its loss.

One year before Lindsay graduated; Kathie and I began the arduous task of looking at new programs. At that time, Michigan special education students had been quite fortunate in that public school programs were available up to the age of twenty-six. (Recently there have been conversations pointed to changing the age limit to twenty-one.) Lindsay truly benefited from those extra years. Now that she was leaving the realm of public schools, however, the programs we considered paled in comparison. It was one disappointing visit after another. There was a sheltered workshop in which clients had their own little workspace and performed jobs that required concise fine motor skills. Also, many of these clients were able to eat their lunches without assistance and even use the vending machines.

There was supervision at every level, but basically in the form of a watchful eye. Most of these people could function at a higher level than Lindsay, and I knew it would not be an appropriate placement.

There were several similar programs that we observed, and Kathie and I were beginning to wonder if there was, indeed, a fit for Lindsay anywhere out there. Then we investigated a few programs in which the clients received close supervision. I knew that Lindsay would not qualify for a one-on-one aide, but we needed a program where there were small groups and several aides available to help out. We discovered programs where the clients were severely multiply impaired, like Lindsay, however they were basically warehoused throughout the day. Lindsay needed action and stimulation. This type of programming was definitely not in Lindsay's best interest.

"This seemingly wonderful program was anything but that. Kathie reported that Lindsay was basically strapped into her wheelchair all day and so was Robbie."

After a few more phone calls, we found a program in Canton that seemed like a good fit. Kathie, Carol Kaczander (Robbie's mother), and I went for a visit to size the program up. We were shown around the facility by very friendly and informative people. The employees were proud of their program, and there was a wide variety of activities for the clients. They had a music room where people were listening to the piano being played, a sensory stimulation room, a gardening center, and even their own resale shop where clients actually worked for part of the day. And, of course, there were community-based experiences such as trips to the mall, restaurants, bowling, and the movies. It *seemed* like a good program for Lindsay and Robbie. So, arrangements were made, transportation was settled, and they were both slated to begin in July. Kathie and I decided that we would drop in the first couple days just to show Lindsay and Robbie a familiar face and to ensure that the transition went smoothly. Kathie visited the first day and I went the next.

This seemingly wonderful program was anything but that. Kathie reported that Lindsay was basically strapped into her wheelchair all day and so was Robbie. She also noticed that there were several clients walking around the facility unsupervised, which could have been a recipe for disaster. At that point in time, Lindsay was still using her walker quite efficiently. It could have been a problem if Lindsay walked around the room and met up with someone who was not observant of her small stature. One slight push and she would have landed on the floor. During lunch time she was not taken out of her wheelchair to sit at a table and, rather than letting her use utensils, the staff fed her. Lindsay has always sat at a table and, with minimal supervision, fed herself. Kathie was dismayed; I was horrified.

Immediately, I called Carol and told her about the situation. We told her that Jeffrey and I were going to observe the next day. Needless to say, we were very anxious. Kathie decided to come along as well, and we thought that it would be a good idea to observe until lunch and then conference. Kathie stated that she was never approached by any of their staff the entire time she visited. There were no introductions or even questions for her. She could have just walked in off the street for all they seemed to care. This completely unnerved Jeffrey and me. We'd thought Lindsay and Robbie would feel safe and enjoy their day in this new setting. We were so wrong. The three of us went to lunch to discuss the problem. We all agreed to withdraw Lindsay from the program and felt certain that Carol would agree as well. Thus ended Lindsay's first experience in a post-graduate program.

It was back to the drawing board. Kathie and I decided to take another look at the Easter Seals program in Bloomfield Hills. We had visited the school over a year before, but did not truly consider it since we heard they were experiencing financial problems and might shut down.

Apparently, they had restructured and we felt the facility deserved another look. They'd changed administrators and adopted a different name; the program was now called New Gateways. It was housed in an elementary school no longer slated for use, and the facility was shared with another school program as well. (There was plenty of room for both programs.) I immediately felt comfortable when we toured the building. At the time, approximately 80 clients attended and there were a wide variety of activities to engage in during the course of the day. The clients were divided into teams, with captains to organize and initiate activities. They had an art room, a health and beauty room, and a large area that was split up to accommodate the majority of the teams and their activities. Community-based outings were conducted on a regular basis and this was an important element for Lindsay. The group leaders decided on various projects such as collecting clothing for the underprivileged, selling candy to help defray the costs of going to restaurants, and there was even a strong parent group that worked tirelessly to ensure stability and continued growth within New Gateways. The staff appeared to be warm and friendly and we were relieved to say, finally, that this would become Lindsay's new stomping grounds.

As the paperwork was being completed for Lindsay's admission to New Gateways, Jeffrey called On Time Transportation to discuss Lindsay's needs. She would be picked up every day in a van and taken to school and back. We wanted to meet the driver and talk about our concerns. The transportation company agreed to send Lindsay's driver to our house to meet us. The next day, Jerome Randall knocked on the door and it was the start of a love affair that continued for years. We told Jerome that since Lindsay was so petite we would prefer that she sit in the front seat. And that was the coveted spot from which she shared many precious moments with Jerome. He enjoyed talking to Lindsay while they drove. In view of the fact that one of Lindsay's many nicknames is "Good," Jerome started to use a variation of the name, calling her "Goody Good." Every morning, after Jeffrey placed Lindsay in her seat and buckled her in, she would reach over to grab Jerome's arm for an affectionate hug. If Lindsay had a runny nose Jerome would wipe it, and when she was in a bad mood and in desperate need of an attitude adjustment, Jerome could make her smile. He also quickly learned that Lindsay enjoyed a refreshing cup of Coca-Cola on her ride home from New Gateways. One afternoon as they drove home, Jerome poured some Coke into a cup for himself then placed it in the holder. Much to his surprise he watched Lindsay grab the magical mixture and gulp it down. Jerome and Lindsay enjoyed driving together on the highway for four years until Jerome decided it was time for a change of pace. He moved away; but whenever he comes to town he always calls and visits. Lindsay misses her buddy.

Chapter Fourteen

"It was during this trip, however, that Lindsay began to exhibit bouts of pain due to arthritic hips."

Spring Break 2006 signaled a much awaited senior trip to Puerto Vallarta, Mexico for Eli and his friends. Forty students were traveling to the Buena Ventura Hotel along with 20 adult chaperones. Our family was going as well. How could we let these maniacs loose on the streets of Puerto Vallarta without a watchful eye? We were going to enjoy a week in the sun while keeping tabs on the seniors. What a blast!

The days were spent in the pool or at the beach, with the occasional shopping or sightseeing jaunt. The hotel was all inclusive, but after a few days we headed to some of the local restaurants for a refreshing change of pace. The kids didn't miss a beat. After a full day in the sun they were off to the clubs and couldn't wait for another opportunity to drink the night away. (The legal drinking age in Mexico is 18 and the kids relished this "adult" privilege.) I must admit that I was quite happy that Chad decided to accompany us on the trip. He went on these evening excursions with Eli and the crew, which made Jeffrey and me feel more secure—if there really is such a thing for the parent of a teenager. Chad even claimed that he enjoyed Eli's Spring Break more than his own.

It was during this trip, however, that Lindsay began to exhibit bouts of pain due to arthritic hips. For years we had known her hips were displaced and that arthritis was compounding the problem. In cold weather she would hesitate while walking as if to regain some sort of composure before taking another step. She also began to draw her right leg up off the ground and balance on her left leg. I don't know how she maintained this pose for what seemed like minutes, but when the pain subsided, her right leg met the pavement once again.

Lindsay used her walker around the house, as well as for short walks outside. It was a rear facing walker that wrapped around her body and was open in the front. This helped with posture, since most people seemed to lean forward in traditional walkers. Lindsay could move with great skill and exhibited fine motor planning while maneuvering around furniture and avoiding door jambs. It was great to watch as she moved about so easily; and it was obvious that she took much pleasure in this. Her most skillful move by far was to lift the walker while standing in place and turn it completely around to walk in the opposite direction. It was as if she only needed a bit of security to actually walk. Before leaving Mexico, however, these delightful times began to decrease and Lindsay only felt comfortable walking when holding onto our hands.

While we were at the resort, we noticed that Lindsay did not want to walk much at all. Then she began to wake up in the middle of the night screaming in pain. This was Chad's signal to pick her up from bed and carry her to another spot in the room to help her relax. We gave her Motrin in addition to Mexican wine. None of these measures appeared to have an effect on the pain. She also had minor outbreaks of discomfort during the day. For these, simply changing her position seemed to alleviate the difficulty.

Upon our return, we called Marty Levinson to fill him in on the situation. He advised us to make an appointment with Dr. Ira Zaltz, an orthopedic surgeon. We managed to get an appointment the very next week. After reviewing x-rays, Dr. Zaltz informed us there was little or no cartilage in the left hip and the right one looked even worse. He recommended that we continue with a regimen of ibuprofen and physical therapy. After a bit of conversation in his office we discovered that he lived around the block and that he even recognized us from our power walks through the neighborhood. (Actually, I am the one powering while Lindsay enjoys the scenery in her wheelchair.) Dr. Zaltz seemed truly interested in Lindsay's problem, yet, at this point, appeared to be conservative in his treatment. I suppose that we were looking for an instant fix to the problem.

Marty also knew of a progressive physical therapist who used nontraditional methods. So we made an appointment to see Peter Kuglin, who worked at Total Body Rehabilitation in Southfield, for an evaluation. We'd heard that it was difficult to get on his "hit" list; nevertheless Peter fit us into his packed caseload. Lindsay was quite reluctant at first when he attempted to manipulate her body. His approach was different from most therapists—he was completely hands on, no machines. Peter also discussed the importance of the osteopathic methodology. We were familiar with this technique from Dr. Goodheart.

By the time our first visit took place, Lindsay had stopped walking completely. Peter definitely had his work cut out for him. Under his care, Lindsay slowly began to walk again, with assistance, but she no longer had interest in using her walker. I believe that she lost confidence. Plus, those arthritic hips were still quite problematic. No matter how much progress Lindsay made with Peter, the pain persisted.

After approximately nine months of therapy and several more appointments with Dr. Zaltz, it was time for some more advanced medical intervention. We had asked for cortisone injections and Marty made a case for this as well. Dr. Zaltz was kind enough to squeeze Lindsay into his tight schedule. Her first set of injections were done on an outpatient basis at William Beaumont Hospital in Royal Oak. According to protocol, Lindsay waited patiently with an IV in her arm, lying on a gurney, for several hours before she was called. Then Jeffrey and I waited in the family area. When Dr. Zaltz appeared twenty minutes later, he told us that all was well. He said that we should see a difference in about a week and to call to him at home to report on her progress. Dr. Zaltz also added that only four injections of cortisone could be used within a year.

Much to our delight, a few days later, we saw a significant difference in Lindsay. She could get out of bed effortlessly and actually walk smoothly around the house. Getting in and out of the car was no longer a problem since her legs weren't stiff and she could manage the movement without pain. She appeared to be pain free—there were no complaints and no more screaming. This was definitely the miracle drug we'd prayed for and we hoped that its effects would last indefinitely.

"For the time being, Lindsay continued to receive much needed relief from the injections, but when the pain reoccurred, she was prescribed Vicodin."

However, our joy was short lived when, a few months later, the beauty of the cortisone appeared to subside. It was back to the drawing board—and to Beaumont Hospital —for another round of bilateral hip injections. This time the relief lasted longer—approximately four glorious months. Lindsay was happy again and we were, too. It's quite difficult, to say the least, when your child is in pain and there's little you can do to help. The situation was even more devastating since Lindsay looked to us to make the pain go away. With each round of injections, Dr. Zaltz did his best to see Lindsay again as quickly as possible.

Since Lindsay has a high threshold for pain, we suggested that the injections be performed at his office instead of the hospital. We explained that, ultimately, it would be in Lindsay's best interest to have the injections done quickly, without the tedious wait as an outpatient. So, in his office, we witnessed her third set of injections. The needle was long and we watched as it entered her hip from the front of her leg. Ultrasound was employed to locate the exact spot for injection. Lindsay let out a bit of a scream from the first injection and then it was the anticipation of the second shot that gave her some fear. But it was over quickly and Lindsay was soon all smiles.

Dr. Zaltz warned us that the shots would eventually stop working, that they were a swift but temporary fix to a complicated problem. He suggested that we consider hip replacement. We were horrified at the proposition. How could Lindsay endure such an intricate surgery and go through physical therapy, only to do it all over again since both hips were affected? Jeffrey and I balked at the idea. We began to investigate alternative, noninvasive measures. In truth, we feared for her life while undergoing such a delicate surgery.

For the time being, Lindsay continued to receive much needed relief from the injections, but when the pain reoccurred she was prescribed Vicodin. We proceeded with caution when administering this drug, resorting to it only infrequently.

Chapter Fifteen

"Mark's family believes he was the oldest person in the world with MSS. He was 19."

It was the Fourth of July, 2007, and I was in the kitchen, as usual. Chad was on the computer, as usual, and he called out, "Hey, Mom, come here. You have to see this." I casually walked into the computer room in anticipation of an interesting tidbit of information. Chad is constantly finding intriguing articles and, in this, he did not disappoint.

A news video from Minnesota. It concerned a young man who was just diagnosed with Marshall-Smith Syndrome. He shared similar features with Lindsay and it was reported that he'd had forty surgeries in his short life. I watched in amazement as his parents talked about his accomplishments with sign language and learning to ride a bike that was adapted for people with disabilities. I could totally relate to the excitement of these precious moments. Mark Arimond's father stated that when he watched his son take off on his bike it was similar to the elation one might experience upon being admitted to Harvard. Most people cannot identify with this statement, but I knew exactly what he meant, and his words were profound.

I have experienced this joy with Lindsay as well as with the boys. Nothing can feel better than when your child reaches a milestone in development, even if, in Lindsay and Mark's case, it occurs years past the expected time. Every accomplishment for our children is exhilarating.

Then the best part of the news clip played. Since there was so little information concerning MSS, Mark's family believed that he was the oldest person in the world with MSS. He was nineteen. Chad looked at me, I returned the gaze, and then we both looked at Lindsay and laughed. I said, "They don't know Lindsay yet!" At the time Lindsay was twenty-seven. Immediately I asked Chad to locate the news station in order to find the Arimonds' phone number. I had never spoken to another parent whose child had MSS. The prospects were so very exciting.

I reflected back to a time when Lindsay was eight years old. Her pediatrician, Marty Levinson, talked to a geneticist at a medical conference who had direct information concerning Marshall-Smith Syndrome. Marty provided me with the telephone number of a family whose child was diagnosed with MSS. It turned out to be a disappointing phone call. The mother was very friendly and we shared information; however, she believed that her child had been misdiagnosed and did not share many of the physical features so common in children with MSS. I was happy for her and hoped that her assessment was correct. Sad to admit, but a part of me believed that she was in denial because I so badly wanted another person to commiserate with after all of those years. Nonetheless, it was a huge disappointment; I was still left in the dark with no one to talk to who could share my grief. As the phone conversation came to a close, we said that we would share pictures, but that never happened. Once again, the sparse literature on Marshall-Smith Syndrome had its hold on me.

As the years passed, however, and the business of life continued, those haunting words of a short lifespan for Lindsay gradually crept to the back of my mind. It's easy to dwell on the negative. The difficulty lies in maintaining a realistic and somewhat positive outlook.

Surprisingly, I received a rather quick response from the news station. And they were more than happy to forward the Arimonds' cell and home numbers. I was still in a bit of shock. I looked at the news clips several more times and once again saw the strong resemblance to Lindsay. It was an eerie feeling. After I received their phone numbers, it took me about a week to actually call them. I couldn't quite reconcile myself to the fact that there were people out there, somewhere, who shared my life, though to what degree I was unsure. Nonetheless, I finally made the phone call.

After a great deal of contemplation about how to begin the conversation—I stumbled through an introduction and told Beth Arimond that I had viewed the news clip about Mark—I proceeded to tell her about Lindsay and she was overjoyed to know that Lindsay was doing well and that she was older than Mark. We shared stories concerning tracheostomies, eating habits, sleep patterns (or lack of them), communication, surgeries, social development, school programs, respite, and the list went on and on. We chatted about every facet of our children's lives and all of the important events that had transpired.

It was exciting, hopeful, and yet bitter-sweet at the same time. Beth told me that since Mark had been diagnosed she had been in contact with several other families through MAJIC, an organization for people with rare conditions. It was absolutely wonderful to finally "make contact" with another family after 27 years. I had absolutely resigned myself to the fact that I would never meet or speak with anyone whose family member had Marshall-Smith Syndrome. Those assumptions were now erased and it felt liberating to finally break the barrier. After our initial conversation, Beth and I spoke every few months. We basically shared family events and kept each other updated on Lindsay and Mark's health and daily routines.

"It was remarkable to think that only a short while ago I knew no one else with Marshall-Smith Syndrome and now there was a network of people to contact across the globe."

In March, 2008, Beth called me with unbelievable news. She told me there was a web site from the Netherlands and it was directed at people with Marshall-Smith Syndrome. Apparently, a family coordinated this site and was looking for other people with MSS to log in and send pictures and information concerning affected family members. Finally there was a global connection. It makes a lot of sense that a young couple would pursue this endeavor. Today, technology joins people together in a myriad of ways—assuming that one possesses the knowledge or hires someone to create a web site. Henk-Willem Laan and his wife, Lisbeth, had the desire to locate others who were born with MSS, and they embarked on a journey to help their son, Joas. I'm sure that they were devastated with the initial diagnosis of their son and they leapt into action.

I was amazed when I logged onto the web site and actually saw the pictures of several children with MSS. There was even a family communication page; however, it was not easily accessed. I wrote about Lindsay and then the information was shared with Sonja Bracke and her husband, Karel. Their daughter, Nina, was twelve years old at the time and they had only met the Laans and Adriana Godani and her parents, Sergio and Ana, several years prior to the development of the web site. I can only imagine that each family felt alone, isolated, and bewildered by this frightful condition.

No two children share the same characteristics. There is a broad spectrum of development, or lack thereof. Every child with MSS is born with their own personal spectrum of difficulties. The common bond in this syndrome is the fact that they all have advanced bone age, similar physical features, and a certain degree of developmental delay. The majority of children also have a compromised airway; however, when treated properly with either a tracheostomy or a nasal pharyngeal tube (a flexible tube that is placed in the nasal cavity and then enters the airway to help with respirations while sleeping), the child can breathe. Once they get past childhood their airways mature, enabling them to have the devices removed. However, there were still some cases reported where the removal of the trach was not successful and it had to be used once again for an indefinite period of time. There was no choice when this occurred: it's a matter of life or death. (Besides having to suction the secretions from the trach to enable the lungs to be clear, the hardest part to deal with in this endeavor is the fact that you can no longer hear your child's voice. Lindsay has never been able to talk; however, with the trach in place, I could not even hear her make sounds, laugh, or cry.)

Within the next few months I received several emails from other families. Everyone could find a thread of similarity with each story. I was still in awe and it was really amazing to know that MSS was a nondiscriminatory condition. It crossed over the boundaries of race, religion, and gender. Its hostages came from all over the world and yet there were only 21 people reported with MSS at that time. I'm sure there are still children who go undiagnosed; however, that number remains astoundingly small.

Interestingly, there was a family from Israel whose daughter had MSS. I couldn't help but think that the likelihood of there being two Jewish families—out of 21 total cases worldwide—was unbelievable. Chad did the math and calculated that the chances of this occurring were one in 250 million. It's hard to wrap your head around that number. It was difficult enough to absorb it when Lindsay was born in 1979, back when it was estimated that her case was one in a million.

On the web site, I discovered that there was going to be a medical conference in the Netherlands, centering around the theme: Rare Disease Day. Our family had just traveled to Israel to visit Todd and Chana Tova during the winter break and, ironically, we had a 12 hour layover in Amsterdam. At that time we had no idea there were three families living in the area whose children had MSS. It was just two short months later that we heard about the web site. Unfortunately, the notion of traveling back to the Netherlands was not on our radar, due to distance and cost. We simply figured that we would hear about all of the details after the conference.

During this time period, Todd and Chana Tova were expecting their first child, our first grandchild. Jeffrey and I were elated at the prospects of becoming grandparents. However, I suffered silently the pangs of fear from years prior when I was pregnant with the boys. Once again I focused on the positive and prayed constantly for a healthy baby. This time my mantra was to be granted a healthy grandchild with no diseases, conditions, or syndromes. I must have repeated that phrase thousands of times and I can only imagine the fear that Todd and Chana Tova had as well. But the glorious day of Shoshana Leiba's birth came on October 3rd, 2008, and she is a beautiful, healthy baby. We were ecstatic as well as relieved. I suppose that this will be the regimen for every one of our future grandchildren.

Todd and Chana Tova had decided to come back to the United States to have their baby. So, as we traveled to New York to welcome our new grandchild into this world, the thought of the Netherlands grew quite remote. During this wonderful visit, my mind was focused only on my growing family and thoughts of the MSS web site were definitely on the back burner.

However, shortly after Todd returned to Israel, I received a surprising email. I was at school and began to read my mail, as usual, during my preparation hour. Everything is generally school related, except for some spam that sneaks in occasionally. At first glance I thought I was seeing things. The name Sonja Bracke was on my school computer. What was this, and how did she get my school email address? I never gave it to her. I was very curious and I opened it with trepidation.

The email read:

Hope you remember us. We had some contact with you in 2008. At the end of February 2009 the MSS Event will take place. We want to invite you to come to the event, with Lindsay, of course, if she is able to travel. We have had enough money sponsored to pay for three tickets for you, if you want to come. It is also possible to stay longer after the event. The costs for the apartment are very low. Maybe you can email me your phone number, then I'll try to phone you and tell you in my best English more about it.

Kind regards,

Sonja Bracke
Also kind regards from Henk-Willem Laan
MSS Research Foundation

I kept looking at the monitor and rereading the letter. I wanted to go out in the hallway and scream for joy—and I certainly would have, were classes not in session. I immediately called Jeffrey and gave him the news. He was just as amazed as me and said "So I guess we're going." However, as much as we desired to take the trip, there was still the "little" problem of getting the red light from my principal since I would be taking several days off from teaching. I emailed Sonja and expressed my gratitude for the tickets and told her that I would have to let her know after I spoke with Dennis McDavid, my building principal, and Bill James, the director of CASA (Center for Advanced Studies and the Arts) where I teach in the afternoon. Sonja replied, "I will light a candle tonight and say a prayer that you will come."

Now, Dennis and Bill are very nice people and understanding as well. I thought this invitation would be a no-brainer, but when dealing with a school and the politics involved, one can never assume anything. I spoke with Bill first and he was elated at the proposition. Bill knew that I had to discuss the situation with Dennis. After a few days of trying to get an appointment, I was able to sit down with him and lay out the entire trip. I provided Dennis with background information about Lindsay and MSS. He sat and listened and then told me that he thought it should work out by taking days off for family related health issues as the conference was about her medical condition. Dennis then had to discuss the matter with the assistant superintendent who, thankfully, also gave her approval.

Chapter Sixteen

"After 28 years we were finally at the threshold of enlightenment."

The idea that I was finally going to meet people with MSS and their parents was absolutely mind blowing. I couldn't believe that this event was actually coming to fruition. I guess I had become comfortable in being alone and now there were going to be nine families present at the conference. This was to be the trip of a lifetime. After 28 years we were finally at the threshold of enlightenment.

As we prepared for the trip we kept receiving emails concerning the format of the conference and pictures of the Kindervallei, where we would be staying. The conference was to be held in Valkenburg aan de Geul, at a Ronald McDonald House. However, when I looked at the accommodations on YouTube, I saw that this was no ordinary facility. First of all, it was built by the renowned artist and architect, Friedensreich Hundertwasser. He wanted to provide families with a unique and pleasant experience. Trust me, he did not disappoint. It was noted that "in this colorful building no door is or estimates the same, no straight line to confess and on the roof and from the wall trees and plants are growing." This facility was designated for respite and it was not affiliated with a hospital.

The primary function of the Kindervallei was for families of disabled children to enjoy a vacation in a warm and uplifting atmosphere. The cost of each apartment was nominal, thus making it accessible to all families. Vibrant colors—oranges, reds, yellows, and blues—surrounded the outside of the building as well as the interior. Even the apartments looked colorful with a variety of different tiles on the walls in the kitchen and the bathroom. The facility was barrier free and, as such, it could accommodate any special needs. There were even tepees on the grounds that could be used in warm weather for a special treat. It is obvious that a great deal of thought and creativity went into the planning and execution of this building. Families of disabled children could vacation in an amazing setting and feel completely comfortable thanks to the unique touches. And with other families present, visitors know that they are accepted and don't have to deal with the stares and lack of accessible equipment that's usually the norm.

As Sonja and I were discussing the conference via email, I had asked her how she found my email address at Berkley High School. Sonja had not heard from most of the families in the United States and she figured that all of the emails either hadn't been accessed or had gone undelivered. So she simply Googled my name and, low and behold, found the link. Isn't technology amazing? Sonja's hope was to find me at work and that the email would finally go through. Her assumptions were correct and her perseverance paid off. As it turned out, we were the only family embarking on this journey from the U.S.

And as we made our preparations it occurred to me that I had read an article many years ago about taking a trip to Holland. It wasn't the typical travel related article; instead, it concerned the experience of raising a child with a disability. The article was written in 1987 and Marty Levinson had given it to me. I remember smiling and crying at the same time as I read Emily Perl Kingsley's beautifully crafted article. It was eloquent and gave voice to an army of mothers who felt exactly like Emily. Her son was born with Down syndrome in 1974. The article reads:

When you're going to have a baby, it's like planning a fabulous trip—to Italy.

You buy a bunch of guide books and make your wonderful plans. The Coliseum. The Michelangelo David. The gondolas in Venice. You may learn some handy phrases in Italian. It's all very exciting.

After months of eager anticipation, the day finally arrives. You pack your bags and off you go. Several hours later, the plane lands. The stewardess comes in and says, "Welcome to Holland."

"Holland?!?" you say. "What do you mean Holland?? I signed up for Italy! I'm supposed to be in Italy. All my life I've dreamed of going to Italy."

But there's been a change in the flight plan. They've landed in Holland and there you must stay.

The important thing is that they haven't taken you to a horrible, disgusting, filthy place, full of pestilence, famine, and disease. It's just a different place.

So you must go out and buy new guide books. And you must learn a whole new language. And you will meet a whole new group of people you would never have met.

It's just a different place. It's slower paced than Italy, less flashy than Italy. But after you've been there for a while and you catch your breath, you look around ... and you begin to notice that Holland has windmills ... Holland has tulips, Holland has Rembrandts.

But everyone you know is busy coming and going from Italy ... and they're all bragging about what a wonderful time they had there. And for the rest of your life, you will say "Yes, that's where I was supposed to go. That's what I had planned."

And the pain of that will never, ever, ever, ever go away ... because the loss of that dream is a very, very significant loss.

But ... if you spend your life mourning the fact that you didn't get to Italy, you may never be free to enjoy the very special, the very lovely thing ... about Holland.*

On February 26th, 2009 we boarded the plane and headed for Holland. We were going to see the windmills, the Rembrandts, and possibly the tulips if the weather permitted. Our family was on an adventure that we never thought possible. I knew there were 21 people with MSS in the world; however, the idea of meeting any of them had seemed quite beyond my expectations. I had seen the children's pictures on the web site and now we were actually going to meet them in person—how completely mind blowing! I wondered, too, how Lindsay was going to react. I wondered how all of us were going to react. It was exciting and frightening at the same time.

It took approximately nine hours to fly to Amsterdam. We watched movies on the airplane and Lindsay ate and relaxed. (I always bring goodies for the family on every trip.) The highlight of any flight with Lindsay is taking her to the bathroom. Those tiny stalls are not comfortable for one person, let alone two, yet Lindsay and I manage quite well. Because of the loud noise created by the airplane, I can't hear if Lindsay actually goes to the bathroom as there's no water in the bowl. So, before Lindsay sits on the toilet I put a lot of toilet paper in that huge bowl and when it changes color I know that our mission has been accomplished. Now, I could just ask her, but there are times when she does not respond and I don't want to take any chances. Just to be safe, I always carry extra clothing.

When we arrived at the Schiphol airport in Amsterdam, Sonja's brother, Edwin, picked us up. He generously volunteered to drive us to Valkenburg, which is about two hours north of the airport. Edwin had to attach a "trolley" to the back of his car to accommodate our luggage. We Americans are notorious for traveling with too much luggage and Edwin came prepared. Without the trolley, we would have been unable to take our belongings with us to the conference.

---

* "Welcome to Holland" by Emily Perl Kingsley, Copyright by EPK, All rights reserved, Reprinted by permission of the author.

Europeans laugh at our over-packing and the use of such large suitcases. I admit we are quite a sight, but I just can't envision traveling with less—especially when traveling with Lindsay. However, when we are schlepping those suitcases from the car to a taxi or to our lodgings, I definitely prefer the European style of travel.)

Edwin was a friendly guy and we certainly connected well. He talked about the Netherlands and its declining economy, which we could all relate to. I asked him if he thought that Lindsay looked like Nina, his niece. I suppose that it wasn't fair to ask such a question, but I was curious. After all, children with MSS share many of the same physical features. Edwin didn't really reply with words, he just sort of shrugged his shoulders and made a grimace.

It took us longer than we expected to arrive at our destination. (We got lost a few times along the way, but I didn't mind since the scenery was so beautiful.) We all recognized the building as we approached—we'd fawned over the pictures so often. The bright colors called out, enticing us to drive up and stay for a while. The color scheme almost reminded me of the 70s and the psychedelic paintings of Peter Max.

I got out of the car and looked around. We all needed to stretch, including Lindsay. She quickly swung her legs around so that we could help her out of the car. It was time to meet her "cousins." Chad came up with that line one day as we were looking at pictures on the MSS web site. There are so few children with this condition and they are definitely connected, just like family members.

I must admit I felt a bit of anxiety as we entered the building. The media was onsite, but that wasn't the part that bothered me. I was about to meet children who were just like Lindsay and shared a huge part of her life. I was also going to meet the parents of these children, and for the first time in 29 years I could speak directly to people who knew exactly how I felt. It was truly liberating to walk through those doors and greet Sonja and Henk-Willem. After all, I had seen their pictures in an interview of the families during a news show in the Netherlands that was comparable to *20/20* or *Dateline*. The only difference was that the entire broadcast was in Dutch. I listened and watched attentively and innately knew the nature of the conversation. Their story was my story as well.

The atmosphere was friendly and the air was filled with contentment. It's as if the entire group was actually saying "at long last." I was completely overwhelmed and on the verge of tears. I had to pull myself together so that I could take in the beauty of the moment. I watched as Nina (Sonja's daughter) flitted around welcoming everyone. She immediately took my hand and Lindsay's. What a social butterfly. I marveled at the way she walked and the fact that she did not need assistance like Lindsay. The other Dutch family, the Godonis, were there as well. Ana and Sergio are doting parents. Their daughter, Adriana, who was six years old, reminded me of Lindsay when she was little. Adrianna had the same curly hair and loved to be held by her parents. She used a walker and moved about easily. They greeted us with a kiss—it was so unusual to be kissed on each cheek when we made our introductions. After a while, however, I really enjoyed the double kiss.

Next we were introduced to Kelli Windebank and Alex Williams from the United Kingdom. Kelli's mother also accompanied them on the trip. She is truly involved with her grandchildren. Ella Windebank has MSS and she was seven years old when they made the trip. Grace, their then-four year old is healthy and an active child. Ella is also quite active and her gait seemed so natural. Her parents told us that she did not have any issues with a compromised airway and that, at first; they did not believe that she had MSS. However, even though she was developing nicely, she exhibited the tell-tale characteristics of advanced bone age. Ella does not have expressive language and her parents are concerned about this as well. Ella moved about easily with the grace of a typical seven year old. She enjoyed pushing around a baby carriage and delighted in the fun of the play structure outside. I, too, was delighted to observe her ease in movement. Certainly, there were vast differences in all of the children. Alex commented that he was the same age as Lindsay, twenty-nine. It was strange and yet amusing at the same time.

The Humphreys, Tom and Olivia, came with their son Adam who was 21 years old. They are also from the United Kingdom. Adam was in a wheelchair and looked like a sturdy young man. He is currently living in a group home since it became quite difficult for Tom to lift and transfer him. Adam had surgery when he was small due to a hole in his spine. He could not sit up without falling over. A rod was placed in his spine and this relieved many problems. Adam sported a red shirt that was really hysterical, proclaiming in bold letters, "I Am Not A Working Person." Tom told us that the group home employees bought Adam the shirt.

Later in the day, the last of the contingent from the United Kingdom arrived. Matthew, 13, was also in a wheelchair. He loves his younger brother and it was apparent that the feeling was mutual. Matthew also displayed a deep interest in a toy drum that he kept on his lap. He truly enjoyed playing the drum throughout the day. His parents, Sara Kironde and Adrian Strain, spoke of Matthew's education and the fact that he lives away at school. They told me that it was a very difficult decision to make, but that it was in Matthew's best interest. They also commented that there were no schools in the vicinity of their home that could educate Matthew properly. He was making advancements and that was worth the pain in the decision making process. Matthew had a great smile and enjoyed all of the action as well.

Raefaela and her mother, Sabrina Fontes da Silveira, traveled from Brazil. Sabrina's friend, Aline Varga de Almeida, accompanied them on the trip to help with the language barrier. Sabrina could only speak Portuguese and Aline translated everything to her since she could speak English. Raefaela and Adriana connected immediately. These six year olds had a wonderful time together. They were constantly laughing and playing with each other. Ana, Adriana's mother, also spoke Portuguese, so it was a true fit.

Matteo, another six year old, traveled from France with his parents, Olivier Jean and Nathalie Servier. Matteo kept everyone laughing. He is quite expressive and when he said "oo la la" the entire room lit up. He could walk with assistance and his bubbly personality was extremely enjoyable. Matteo is very conversant as well.

Then we finally got to meet Joas since he'd been taking a nap when we arrived. Joas has blond curly hair and a smile so bright it's contagious. Looking at Joas, he could have been the blond version of Lindsay when she was a baby. It was obvious that all of the children were happy.

Our meals took place in a large dining area making it very easy for everyone to socialize. The families were interested in finding out more information about MSS as well as sharing individual stories with each other. Everyone appeared to feel at ease and took advantage of the time we spent together to make connections. The big questions revolved around diagnosis of MSS and health issues when the children were small.

After such a busy and enlightening day, one might think we should have been exhausted, but that's not the way we operate. When our family travels, we like to make the most of our time. So after dinner we embarked on a short excursion to Maastrict. I had read that it is located on the Maas River and attracts international tourists. It was founded by the Romans and has a rich history. That was enough to entice me. Sonja volunteered to drive us into town. She said that Maastrict was close to Valkenburg and that it would probably take us about ten minutes to get there. When we were dropped off at what appeared to be the center of town, I was in awe of the architecture. The city was beautiful; historic buildings and monuments were everywhere. We walked around, taking in the sights. After stopping at an outside café for a snack, we decided to hail a cab since we had been up for approximately 36 hours. Still, it was so nice to be outside and enjoy the weather at the end of February. We could never do this back at home in Michigan!

Chad found us the perfect cab. A throwback to the 70s, it was decorated with colorful flowers. The driver gave us a brief history of Valkenburg and Maastrict. I asked about the flower power cab and he told us that his boss was an old hippie.

When we returned to the Kindervallei, there were still several families talking casually. Very shortly, most decided to retire since Saturday was going to be a full day of presentations from Dr. Raul Hennekam and Dr. Adam Shaw. There was also going to be a discussion by Dr. Inge van Balkam, who was presenting psychological features. Dr. Hennekam is originally from the Netherlands and he diagnosed Nina, Adriana, and Joas. In the interim Adam, Ella, and Matthew were seen by his team. They had been conducting research on Marshall-Smith Syndrome and the results of their findings were to be presented to the group. Everyone was quite anxious to hear the most recent information.

"Even though many of us already knew the various congenital anomalies, they became more concrete due to the studies completed in England. Now there was a basis of comparison with ten MSS children."

On Saturday morning we all had breakfast together before the conference began. The food was quite interesting and different from what we were used to. Since Jeffrey is an early riser, he naturally was in the main dining room talking with a few of the parents. As the rest of us were getting ready, he came back to the apartment. "You're not going to like the food," he said. "Hopefully Lindsay can find something to eat." He said there was plenty of wonderful, freshly baked bread, a wide variety of cheese, and a beef dish to complement the meal. It all sounded great—if we were going to be eating lunch or dinner—but Lindsay and I chose good old cereal instead.

After breakfast we were all told to enter the conference room for the presentations. The media was there again to listen to the speakers and then talk with us. They were very interested in this rare condition and they wanted the public to be aware as well. In setting up the web site, one of Henk-Willem's goals was to garner public attention to rare diseases and to start a foundation that could help with research. In the short time since its inception, the foundation was able to raise over 40,000 Euros for research and to sponsor the medical conference.

Henk-Willem, Lisbeth, and Sonja organized an amazing event. To begin with, the accommodations were wonderful. Apparently Sonja, Karel, and Nina had been at the Kindervallei several times and they suggested that it would be a perfect site for the event. Next, all of the meals were prepared by local chefs who gave us the true flavor of the Netherlands. And the pastries were absolutely delectable. Every detail was covered so that all of the families could just be comfortable, share information with each other, and enjoy the time we had together.

Since Raul Hennekam speaks English, Dutch, and French, the information he imparted was easily understood by this international group. Aline was able to translate in Portuguese for Sabrina as well. There was even a Dutch translator on the stage and every sentence was repeated for those in the crowd who only spoke this language.

Dr. Hennekam began the forum by discussing the various syndromes that share similarities with MSS. He then showed pictures of these children so we could discern the close connection that all of these diseases have in common. Some of the syndromes include Weaver, Soto's, Ehlers-Danlos Type III, and Stickler syndrome, to mention just a few. I knew about two of these conditions and was surprised to find that there were more syndromes that had features in common with those of MSS. Next, the micro-arrays (a grid of DNA segments of known sequence)of blood were shown and these had been analyzed from several of the families. The blood panels did not show any conclusive links. Dr. Hennekam suggested that more people needed to be studied in order to find connections in the blood. Definitely a catch 22. A larger group would unveil more information but, with only 21 known cases, it wasn't possible to assemble a larger group.

The families from the Netherlands and the United Kingdom had all met with Dr. Hennekam and Dr. Shaw in

2008 for examinations and blood work. Even the parents had blood drawn in order to try to find a common denominator for this rare condition. Their destination was the Institute of Child Health at University College London and Great Ormond Street Hospital for Children in London. Here the doctors probed the chromosomal anomalies that many of the children displayed. While it was noted that no two cases of MSS were the same, there was a common link within a range of physical features. After perusing the literature for many years this list of features was not a surprise to me. Dr. Hennekam stated that many of the children have large eyes and may be light sensitive. At times, Lindsay appears to be crying; however, her eyes are tearing due to light exposure. She wears sunglasses to help with this problem and we adjust the light in the house—especially in the morning—so it doesn't cause her to tear. The list continued with features such as small upturned nose, broad forehead, small chin, advanced bone age, blue sclerae (blue coloring in the whites of the eyes), respiratory problems, developmental delay, failure to thrive, abnormalities of the fingers ... and the beat goes on. After a while this information was truly depressing to hear since so many of those features applied to our child.

On a refreshing note, it was asserted that there were no repeat cases reported in the literature thus far. I carried the information one step further by telling the group that Jeffrey and I became proud grandparents to a healthy baby girl in October of 2008. I knew this information was encouraging for the families.

Then Dr. Shaw continued the presentation with information that was gathered from the ten families who'd participated in the study. He stated that of the ten children studied, breathing problems were evident in eight of them. The study consisted of four males and six females. There were eye problems in six of the ten children such as glaucoma, small optic nerves, large eyes, and nearsightedness. Other areas of interest were the hands and feet. There were deep creases in both, and the large toe on each foot appeared to look like a finger since it was so long. In some cases the nails on the hands were wider than usual and protruded to the sides of the finger. There was a lack of mobility seen in the hands as well. The teeth and gums were swollen in a few of the children and irregular teeth were also found in the mouth. Dr. Shaw stated that scoliosis was present in five of the ten by age seven, and it was severe in two cases. In terms of mobility, he said that walking was generally delayed and many never walked but crawled. In conclusion, Dr. Shaw and Dr. Hennekam stressed that airway obstruction can be a long-term problem and in Europe NPA airways (nasal pharyngeal) were preferred to tracheostomy. It was also stressed that jaw surgery may be effective in relieving airway issues. They suggested that anesthesia should be safe in experienced hands with appropriate precautions.

It certainly was a lot to absorb.

Even though many of us already knew the various congenital anomalies (birth defects), they became more concrete due to the studies completed in England. Now there was a basis of comparison with ten MSS children. Many health concerns were identified and remedies presented. Of course, there was the ever looming question of lifespan. A great number of the children present, however, had already surpassed the highest age mentioned in the older literature, which was between two and three years old. Nina was 13, Matthew 14, Adam 21, and Lindsay was 29 at the time of the conference. All of those present were thrilled to hear that Lindsay was healthy and "an old lady." They were even more elated to see her in person. She gave hope for their children and there's nothing that can top that.

After several more speakers, there was a break for lunch. A journalist from the local newspaper, *The Trouw*, wanted to interview our family. We discussed all of the background information concerning Marshall-Smith Syndrome and how we discovered the web site that led us to the Netherlands. The reporter was interested in Lindsay's daily routine and health issues as well. When he finished the interview he took our email address and said that he would send us a copy of the article and picture. Lindsay was now a celebrity.

The remainder of the day was spent talking with the doctors on an individual basis. When Dr. Hennekam approached us at lunch, we wanted to apprise him of Lindsay's hip problems; particularly the severe arthritis. Jeffrey and I told him that for the past two years she had been receiving injections of cortisone in both hips. These had worked very well in relieving pain and helped Lindsay to walk. However, we noticed that the duration of such relief was diminishing and the injections were required more frequently. We also discussed the fact that her orthopedic surgeon, Dr. Zaltz, stated that eventually she would need hip replacement surgery. Dr. Zaltz was fantastic in accommodating us whenever Lindsay was in pain but, as of late, he gently reintroduced the subject again discussing the long term benefits.

Dr. Hennekam said that children with MSS show evidence of a connective tissue disorder. (Jeffrey and I didn't have a clue how this fit in with surgery.) Dr. Hennekam explained that a few of the children with MSS had hernia repairs that did not work due to this disorder. The surgery was repeated several times with the same result. We feared this might happen with a hip replacement. Dr. Hennekam had concerns as well.

Later on, we spoke with Dr. Inge van Balkom, a psychologist. She had been compiling information on many of the children and gathering data based on testing, as well. Dr. van Balkom was interested in the various developmental stages that Lindsay experienced. She had a battery of questions from Lindsay's childhood and we answered to the best of our recollections. Since Lindsay is the oldest person with MSS, Dr. van Balkom wanted to gather as much information as possible. All of the findings would be instrumental in evaluating and helping other people with MSS.

The remainder of the conference was spent talking and sharing with the families. Most of us related stories concerning our children's medical history, progress in specific areas, anxiety issues, and just daily living experiences with a child who has a rare condition. It seemed so natural to be able to talk with these families. We walked outside a lot since the grounds were lovely. On Sunday, the kids even enjoyed a petting farm that was organized by Henk-Willem and Sonja. After a quick view of the animals Jeffrey, Lindsay, and Chad decided to take a train to Maastrict for more sightseeing adventures. The rest of the dads and their children decided to stay close to the Kindervallei.

The ladies, however, went to a spa. All of the "mums" participated and it was a relaxing, indulgent experience. We drove to a very old hotel that had been completely renovated. To me, it looked like it could have been a palace at one time. There were beautiful gardens surrounding the building. The first step at this wonderful spa was a hand massage, with an application of wax to help alleviate dry skin and smooth the overall appearance of the hands. Boy, I really was in desperate need of this treatment. Then we proceeded to the pool area and selected an herbal wrap for our upper or lower extremities, whichever we desired. The warmth and aroma was extremely gratifying. We all simply relaxed in the moment and chatted by the pool. Some went for a swim and others sat back, absorbed in conversation. Since time is always a precious commodity in my life, I don't treat myself to such luxuries very often. Sonja knew from her own experience with Nina that all of the mums were on a tight schedule. The spa was just what the doctor ordered.

When it came time to depart from the Kindervallei, it was difficult to say goodbye to our new friends. I definitely like to think of them as family now since we all share similar experiences. The nice thing is that no one has to feel cut off any more. I certainly felt like I had been on an island for so many years. Thanks to the Internet, however, we could remain connected. Everyone kissed, the two cheek approach, and hugged. It was difficult not to let the flood gates open. When I said goodbye to Henk-Willem and thanked him for the hundredth time for organizing such an incredible event, he said, "Maybe I will see you in a year, maybe two or even in five years. However long, I will definitely see you again."

We left in high spirits and, of course, our cab driver laughed at the number of suitcases we had in our possession.

As we drove toward the airport, our driver received a call and then told us that we were in the local newspaper. There was a lengthy article and picture as well. He wrote down the name of the paper and he told us to pick it up at the airport.

In our excitement to purchase the newspaper in the terminal, I discovered that I'd left my purse and two other bags in the cab. My purse contained all of our passports and our money. We looked at each other and panicked. Jeffrey told Chad to run outside after the cab to see if the driver had left. He'd told us that he was returning to Valkenburg. However, the driver was nowhere to be seen.

We tried to maintain our composure as we headed for the information kiosk. We explained our situation to the woman working there and stated that we were at a medical conference in Valkenburg. She looked at Lindsay and exclaimed that she had seen her on the news the night before. Lindsay's celebrity status was the key to finding our belongings!

The woman at the kiosk tracked down one of the doctors present at the medical conference, who provided us with the phone numbers necessary to locate our cab. A few phone calls later, she contacted the supervisor of transportation who radioed our driver. The driver said that he would pull to the side of the highway and look for our bags, then call right back. As we waited, the woman translated the news article from Dutch into English, since we didn't recognize a word except for "Lindsay" and "Marshall-Smith Syndrome." The article was accompanied by a large picture of Jeffrey, Nina, and Lindsay.

After a few nervous minutes, we received the good news that all of our belongings were, indeed, in the cab and that the driver was heading back to meet us. When this nice young man arrived, I thanked him profusely. He wished us well, then said, "I'll probably never see you again, but it's been memorable." I certainly won't forget the anxiety of those moments, nor the kindness and honesty of our cabbie.

After all that, we still had some spare time to travel into Amsterdam and explore the city. Once again we were in awe of the architecture and the sense of history. After a few hours we returned to Schiphol airport for our flight, definitely ready to depart. The conference had truly been an amazing experience.

After settling in at home and returning to work, I found the time to email Sonja to tell her about our mishap with the cab. I told her that the article in *The Trouw* was translated by the woman who'd recognized Lindsay. As a matter of fact, when we checked our bags, several of the airport staff said that they had seen the news program concerning the MSS Event. Sonja's response went straight to the point. She commented, "Funny to hear that Lindsay was recognized at the airport. Normally people would not have paid attention or were too afraid to make contact, and now she is a celebrity."

Chapter Seventeen

"At this point we intensified our search for alternate methods to alleviate the pain."

After two years of cortisone injections, Dr. Zaltz suggested that we talk with another doctor in his practice who is an experienced surgeon with knee and hip replacements. We made the appointment reluctantly. Dr. Greene was very friendly and thoroughly explained the surgery, showing us the prosthetic devices that are employed. It was truly interesting and educational. Dr. Greene was impressed with Lindsay's posture, since her x-rays showed a 64-degree curve due to an upper scoliosis. In addition, her gait still seemed to be quite strong. We discussed her airway issues, including the trach she had when she was younger. We also went over the particulars of Marshall-Smith Syndrome, as Dr. Greene was not well acquainted with them. Jeffrey and I asked if Dr. Gilmore could intubate Lindsay if we decided to move forward with the surgery. He didn't have a problem with that. At the end of the appointment, he stated that we would know when it was time for a hip replacement. Perhaps so, but the thought of surgery and the long recovery appeared quite inconceivable.

As the years passed Lindsay's situation changed and, frankly, we were up against the wall. Lindsay's last injections were performed in June 2009 and just two weeks later the pain returned. We thought that we had realized the depth of Lindsay's pain until recently. I went for a walk with her when, seemingly out of nowhere, her legs locked up and she screamed as if someone was torturing her. Then this started to occur when she was sitting, sleeping, or even going to the bathroom. It became totally unpredictable when this extreme pain would strike.

We then intensified our search for alternate methods to alleviate the pain. We were told of a doctor who specialized in sports rehabilitation using noninvasive methods. Naturally, we were intrigued. During our first appointment, we learned that she employed deep muscle massage and manipulation of the T-Band. Lindsay relaxed while receiving these treatments and afterward walked and felt more comfortable. However, the outcome did not last long. We continued with this therapy for several months since Lindsay enjoyed temporary relief, but we expanded our search for other treatments.

We asked several doctors about using the same procedure that's beneficial for knee pain, but they recommended against it. More phone calls led us to Dr. Morris Brown, who heads the pain clinic at Henry Ford Hospital. He informed us that the therapy to reduce knee pain was indeed used in his clinic for hip pain as well. In fact, he emailed us studies that promoted this type of treatment. Since Lindsay's painful bouts were on the increase, Morris helped to set up an appointment at the clinic the very next day. He had informed his colleagues about Lindsay's condition and they were ready for us. After listening to Lindsay's two-year history of pain, they felt that it might be beneficial for her to receive bi-lateral hip injections of Hyalagan once a week for a three week period. Hyalagan is a treatment for osteoarthritis and it comes from a rooster's comb. The results of injecting Hyalagan were not as swift as cortisone, they explained; after the three week period it would require more time to establish proof of effectiveness. With this medicine, however, Lindsay might regain the needed fluid in her hip joints, thus eliminating the pain. The doctors stated that a nerve could be causing problems as well, and this would be another avenue to pursue. In their opinion, hip replacement surgery could be life threatening, given Lindsay's airway predicament. Obviously, Jeffrey and I were pleased that there were still possibilities to explore and we were willing to try any viable alternative. The three-part treatment gave Lindsay an edge for a while: but this band aid lost its adhesive after a few months.

In the interim, debilitating pain became the norm; Lindsay needed something stronger to stave off pain between appointments. We were given Lidocaine patches to place on her hips to help eliminate discomfort. The first day Lindsay seemed to do well with this treatment. After that, however, it was a lost cause. The patches irritated her and, after the second day, we discontinued them. Then, a few days later, Lindsay woke up and could not straighten her legs. They were drawn up tight, as if her knees were locked in place. Lindsay screamed uncontrollably and her face bore the expression of the agony she was experiencing. It was a horrific scene and no matter what we did or said, she found no relief. We gave her some pain medication and tried sitting her up with a pillow behind her back and a phone book on the floor to rest her feet upon. (Since Lindsay's feet don't always reach the floor from a sitting position, the phone book was often employed.) Whatever we tried on that agonizing day did nothing to alleviate the problem. Finally, several hours later, Lindsay was able to stand up and take a few steps. We were all completely wiped out.

It's not a pretty sight when the grown men in the house are reduced to tears. But no one wants to watch Lindsay suffer and they all felt her agony. I witnessed red eyes and faces so forlorn it broke my heart. I knew what they were thinking as well. Lindsay did not deserve this unjust situation in her life. She definitely had enough to deal with already before her hip problems.

When Lindsay experienced pain and looked to us for help, I couldn't stop wondering if she knew that we were trying our best.

Ultimately, I was reminded of a conversation I had with Mark's mother, Beth Arimond. She told me that not a day went by when Mark did not feel pain. I was saddened to hear this. Now I understood Beth's pain as well.

Chapter Eighteen

"When I look into Lindsay's eyes I see a wonderful young lady who will become very confused and upset when Jeffrey and I are not present."

Most parents desire the same things for their children: health, happiness, a good education, and ultimately, independence. When contemplating the future for Lindsay, however, such wishes seem unattainable. Back when Lindsay was a little girl her entire future seemed like a faraway place beyond the realm of possibility. Every year we made birthday plans and, as the special day arrived, I felt grateful to reach that milestone—and fearful it might be the last one. There was also the dread of witnessing Lindsay's developmental progress and the huge gap between her and the other children. Still, I took great solace in knowing that she was here, alive, and I could revel in the fact that Lindsay was beating the odds.

It would be nice to think of Lindsay as an independent woman, capable of taking care of herself and sailing through life with the "normal" problems that most individuals encounter, such as, "Who will I marry?" or "Where do I want to live?" I would love it if Lindsay could contemplate these things. But the fact of the matter is that she simply cannot and will never be able to. My heart aches from this knowledge, and I am powerless to change a solitary thing. When Lindsay does make decisions they are on a much smaller scale. She can decide what color or type of clothing she likes best, what she wants to eat, or whether she wants to go out for a drive somewhere. Independence is a luxury—one that Lindsay will never grasp.

Jeffrey and I know that Todd, Chad, and Eli will be able to provide for themselves. They have graduated from college. They all have a solid work ethic and are able to make decisions that will positively impact their futures. We take a great deal of pride in their accomplishments. But for Lindsay, the future is one that must be created by us. Jeffrey and I have to ensure that Lindsay will be taken care of when we are no longer capable or when we are no longer here.

When I look into Lindsay's eyes I see a wonderful young lady who will become very confused and upset when Jeffrey and I are not present. Loss is difficult for any person, but when your child is severely impaired the impact becomes magnified. I do not want to think about the loneliness, the sorrow, and the utter devastation of this period in Lindsay's life. I can only reflect back to an article I read in the paper many years ago. It described the agony of an impaired man who had recently confronted the death of his mother. He simply stood in the window of their home and awaited her return. There was even a picture of this lost soul as he gazed through the window. At the time, I immediately envisioned Lindsay in this situation and chills began to freeze my soul.

People generally like to think they are indispensable, that no one can take their place. The fact remains there is always someone waiting in the wings to move right in and do the same or even better job. I like to imagine that no one can teach as effectively as I have through the years, but I would be deluding myself. I know I have touched many lives through my teaching, but the beat goes on and the music does not stop for anyone.

However, parents hold a distinctly different position. Their job is never quite finished and they are, in fact, indispensable. If they have been successful, replacement is not an option. The sting of loss is great and the void even greater. I don't have a clone that is 30 years younger than me, ready to fill my shoes and replicate what I have been doing for Lindsay. Yet, I still want the same quality of life for Lindsay that she has grown accustomed to after I'm no longer capable of providing it.

Throughout the years we have broached the subject of Lindsay's future with the boys. I must admit, these conversations have been infrequent, and it's difficult for me to remain composed while discussing the subject. It's delicate and depressing. We have attempted to bring up the subject on a casual basis, when sitting around the dinner table. Todd has stated that he wants to take care of Lindsay when we are no longer capable. He and Chana Tova said they would move back from Israel to help in this situation. Chad and Eli have also expressed interest in living with Lindsay when the time comes. I couldn't ask for better sons. But they are entitled to have their own lives and to pursue their own dreams. This is a huge commitment, one that takes inordinate amounts of time and patience. I'm sure the boys could master all the details and provide for Lindsay, if there was no other alternative, but they are her brothers, not her parents.

Jeffrey and I have talked about JARC (Jewish Association for Residential Care) and the services they provide to people with disabilities. JARC is a non-profit, non sectarian organization founded in 1969 by a group of parents who were concerned about the future of their children with developmental disabilities. We have employed several people from this agency to provide respite care for Lindsay when Jeffrey and I go out on the weekend. The boys always "check out" the caregivers and size up their relationships with Lindsay. Most of the time the employees receive good reviews.

JARC also has a fine reputation for its group homes. Clients can live in condos, apartments, or houses with 24-hour supervision. They are generally placed with people who have similar abilities and interests. Funding comes from the state as well as families. The environment is safe, the employees are caring individuals, and all of the homes instill Jewish values and observe Jewish holidays, as well.

Even with all the accolades they receive, when I think of Lindsay living in a JARC home I become frozen with fear. I know they have a model program but Lindsay can't pick up the phone and tell us that she isn't happy or that the food isn't what she expected. Who will buy her clothes and make sure that she is always fashionable? What about her hair and all of the "beautification" that enables her to look her best? Will she be loved? It makes me feel sick to the core knowing that strangers will be providing her care. I can't envision this day and the floodgates will never close on this discussion. I need to know that Lindsay will be treated with the utmost care, and who is better equipped than her family? It's a dilemma without a resolution—at least at this juncture in time.

As the years move quickly by, Jeffrey and I know too well that we must provide for Lindsay's well-being. This next chapter in life will not be pursued with joy. It's our responsibility to do the very best for our daughter. After all, she deserves a rich and fulfilling life. If we don't make arrangements, who will?

Chapter Nineteen

"I even made a bargain with God"

Dr. Raoul Hennekam, Dr. Adam Shaw, et al., published an extensive article in the *American Journal of Medical Genetics* in November of 2010, which highlighted 19 patients with Marshall-Smith Syndrome. Lindsay has a "feature article" within the publication since she is the oldest person with MSS. There are no frightening pictures, just lovely views of Lindsay as she progressed throughout the years. After interviewing families and gathering data, they discovered that some MSS patients have a similar chromosomal variance. However, not all of the patients exhibit this gene, an indicator that there are still many unknown factors. According to the article, "All definite cases of MSS have occurred sporadically with no familial recurrence or parental consanguinity. MSS is not a genomic disorder." Another interesting fact is that the MSS gene is not produced by either the mother or father. MSS has always been an unknown entity, and now there are some questions answered for all of the families concerned.

All of this information was of interest, however, Lindsay's struggle for pain relief and restored function was not in any of the literature. The Hyalagan injections provided minimal relief, and now a few cortisone injections along the way didn't seem to pack a punch. Next, Oxycontin was prescribed (10 milligrams, twice daily). Combined with Xanax and some Advil, Lindsay appeared to be a bit more comfortable. But then again, there were times when I didn't even know if the drugs were truly working.

Prolotherapy was recommended. This is a series of hip injections that consist of "a simple, natural technique that stimulates the body to repair painful areas when the natural healing process needs a little assistance." A substance is injected into the affected area that basically causes irritation and subsequent healing. Prolotherapy definitely irritated Lindsay and, after a six-week regimen, the treatment was stopped.

So we decided that surgery was probably the next step. At this juncture we needed to have a second opinion in order to make an informed choice. Mike, the husband of Mary Lynn, Lindsay's nurse at Henry Ford Hospital, worked at the University of Michigan and was able to get us an appointment with an orthopedic surgeon who had the reputation of being "The Fixer." He took on difficult and unusual cases. When we arrived, there were x-rays and then we were led to an examination room. When the doctor entered, Jeffrey and I filled him in on all of Lindsay's background information and focused on her current predicament. As he looked at her x-rays, he told us that he did not think that Lindsay had enough bone to hold a prosthetic. He wanted to consult with the orthopedic team at U of M before making any decisions. We were told that he would get back with us shortly. Well, it took two weeks before we heard from his P.A. She repeated the same thing he stated in the exam room—Lindsay did not have enough bone for a successful hip replacement.

Jeffrey and I knew that we had to see Dr. Greene again to discuss this recent information. We were confused and worried. At this appointment, he listened to the entire scenario and seemed unfazed by the information. Dr. Greene then showed us Lindsay's x-rays and proceeded to discuss his strategy with the surgery. He felt comfortable with proceeding and that helped us enormously. He then told us that he would put together a special team and we set the date for July 16, 2010. Dr. Amjad would assist with the intubation to maintain Lindsay's airway and the anesthesiologist was contacted to discuss the particulars of MSS. But before we left his office, we asked Dr. Greene for an injection of cortisone to give Lindsay potential relief before the surgery. It had been six months since her last injection and there was a possibility it just might work.

We had to wrap our heads around this huge event. Rabbis were contacted for blessings and in one of my many conversations with God I told Him that if this was the direction He intended then we were now ready to follow. I felt like Abraham when he was about to sacrifice Isaac on Mount Moriah. That story ends with a wonderful result: life. That is exactly what we wanted; a wonderful life for Lindsay. I even made a bargain with God. I would change some eating habits. According to *Kashruth* (Jewish dietary laws) there should be no consumption of pork or shellfish. I was going to stop eating those delectable bottom feeders, including my favorites: shrimp and lobster. I was also going to eliminate baby back ribs from the menu as well. From now on it would be beef ribs and only fish with scales and fins. Part of the plan was to also pay close attention to Kosher products and use them in our home. I had to give, in order to receive.

A week after Lindsay's appointment she was pain free and walking with our assistance. We were all elated since this was a minor miracle. But we knew that cortisone was only a band aid. Even so, it was wonderful to see Lindsay so joyful. Marty Levinson suggested that we call Dr. Greene and apprise him of the situation, but he was on vacation. When Jeffrey finally spoke to him, it was the day before Lindsay's hip replacement. Dr. Greene stated that Lindsay is high risk and if the cortisone was working, we could make the call to postpone the operation and reschedule when necessary. The surgery was cancelled – we decided to wait.

Unfortunately, after subsequent injections, the pain alleviation diminished. Lindsay's leg muscles atrophied and she even lost weight. She still had a fine appetite, but minimal walking contributed to this problem. She became stiff quite frequently and had to be carried as a result. There was one last alternative out there on the horizon.

After watching *60 Minutes* one Sunday evening, we were mesmerized by the miracles performed by Dr. Anthony Atalla and his research team at the Wake Forest Institute for Regenerative Medicine. We watched a segment concerning the growth of human organs, specifically fingers and bladders. The latter have already been successfully implanted in several people with Spina Bifida. The interviewer commented that Dr. Atalla's work is like something out of a Frankenstein movie. Naturally a light bulb flashed in my mind. If they can create bladders in the lab—then why not cartilage? I contacted his office and Lindsay's name was placed in their database.

So we were at the crossroads once again. Decisions had to be made. We were filled with hope, faith and a positive attitude. We knew that, ultimately, Lindsay would emerge from this fight with a beautiful smile and two feet planted firmly on the ground.

Epilogue

In May of 2011, just before my school year ended, I decided to search the Internet for viable sources of artificial injectable cartilage. Much to my surprise there were many universities and private companies that had been engaged in this type of research for years. I came across an article by Dr. Jennifer Elisseeff from 2003. As I read the article, I saw that there had been progress in this field. So I decided to send an email and discuss Lindsay's condition in hope of a remedy that would ultimately avoid surgery. I have sent many emails throughout the years to researchers and, to my dismay, answers never came. So I naturally thought a response would take a long time, or never happen at all. Much to my surprise, the very next day, one of Dr. Elisseeff's associates responded. I was in shock. His name was Dr. Norman Marcus. His email read:

> I am the orthopedic surgeon who works with Dr. Elisseeff. I have never heard of this particular syndrome, but will be happy to do a search; with such a small number of patients it's unlikely there is much out there. Where do you live?

I responded and was simply grateful that someone was willing to help. After a few short days I heard from Dr. Marcus again. He offered programs that research the genetics of rare diseases, but there was no direct answer to my query. I simply wanted to know if this was a possibility for Lindsay. I sent out another email and then Dr. Elisseeff wrote me back. Another big surprise. She stated:

I forwarded your message to my primary orthopedic collaborator who planned clinical trials (in Europe). He mentioned he may be a little while getting back to you as he wanted to do some research but he is working on it. Best wishes and we will continue to work hard to make something better for you.

These comments were certainly encouraging and I knew we were on the right track. Exactly where it would lead was totally unknown, but we had tread these waters before.

Several months passed and I had yet to hear from this source in Europe. My hopes were beginning to wane, but I held on. In August I emailed Dr. Elisseeff and asked about our discussion. No response. I decided to give it a month; she could be on vacation or very busy. Then I shot her another email and there was no response once again. The school year began and I was immersed in lesson plans, essays, and the usual high school drama. Lindsay's hips were the same; she definitely was not getting any better but had become accustomed to the regimen and knew how to avoid pain with certain movements (or lack thereof). In November, Jeffrey and I made an appointment with Dr. Greene once again and knew that surgery would be the focus of our visit. An x-ray revealed that Lindsay's right hip was fragmented. She was no longer standing on both feet. Her right leg was elevated to avoid pain.

We started taking Lindsay to a new physical therapist since Peter Koughlin left Michigan for a practice in Windsor. Angus Williams of Australian Manual Physical Therapy was now Lindsay's therapist. She would smile and shake her head "yes" in response to my comment, "You're going to see Angus this afternoon." Most times Lindsay would also say her famous "good." They have a wonderful connection and Angus even refers to Lindsay as his "girlfriend." He can usually get Lindsay to say her special words and sometimes we hear Lindsay utter "good girl." That's when you know you're on her "good" side. During most sessions Angus would stretch Lindsay's muscles and attempt to relax her knee and hip through manipulative therapy so she could put weight on her right leg.

Usually his technique worked and Lindsay would extend her leg. It also helped to relieve her pain. However, it was short-lived and she would draw it up again within a day or two. Angus was helping to maintain Lindsay's range of motion and that was no easy task given the deterioration of her hips. When I broached the subject of a total hip replacement with Angus, he only had great reviews of Dr. Greene and stated that everyone's comment after the surgery was, "Why did I wait so long?" I began to wonder this myself.

At this appointment, Dr. Greene asked Lindsay to stand up and she did so readily, just on one leg though. He stated that we would never be able to endure the pain that she had been experiencing. Dr. Greene commented that Lindsay had the potential to walk again and that we really should think about scheduling the surgery. At this point there wasn't a solitary thing to contemplate anymore. Her health wasn't improving, she had lost all of her mobility and, thus, her independence, so it was definitely time to embrace the situation and move forward. Upon leaving Dr. Greene's office I asked Lindsay if she was prepared for a total hip replacement and she nodded her head in agreement: a definitive yes. We were told that the earliest openings for this type of procedure were in March. It seemed like ages away and yet, right around the corner. Jeffrey and I discussed the scenario with Todd and Chana Tova, Chad, and Eli and they were all on board. Everyone had reservations and was fearful, but they knew it was the only step to take in this situation; a step in the right direction.

In the interim, I emailed Dr. Elisseeff one more time. I guess it was a last ditch effort. Once again she did not reply, but Dr. Norman Marcus did. I desperately wanted to know if injectable artificial cartilage was on the horizon and if it could help Lindsay. He asked for my phone number and much to my surprise he called to discuss Lindsay's issues. Jeffrey and I were quite impressed.

Here was a man who did not know us, and yet he took the time to call and impart his wisdom and try to answer our questions. Dr. Marcus told us that he had worked with special needs children in New Mexico and that the only way to solve Lindsay's hip problems was to move forward with the surgery. He stated that, "In a perfect world, if all the stars were aligned properly and there was FDA approval, Lindsay would still not be the first in line for this type of therapy." Athletes, those who are in great physical condition, are the ones who will receive injectable cartilage. Many medical researchers are working on this valuable therapy. Dr. Marcus was honest and forthright. Even though the articles sounded promising, there was much to accomplish in this field and Lindsay was definitely not a candidate. It was another letdown but we were still headed in the right direction once again. This time was different because we irrevocably *knew* there were no other options for Lindsay.

Every time Chad and Eli spoke with Lindsay they would tease her and say that she was going to be the Bionic Woman (ironically, *Lindsay* Wagner played this role in the television series in the 80s). We would all ask her if she was going to receive a new hip and she would just laugh and nod her head in agreement. This became our routine and we thought that Lindsay comprehended the situation with a bit of comedy. That laughter, however, quickly turned to anxiety. After all of the pre-surgical elements were completed (blood, urine, EKG) Lindsay was set to go. We arrived at Beaumont Hospital on March 28th at 5:30 in the morning and pulled in to the parking structure. When we proceeded to place Lindsay in her wheelchair and started walking into the hospital, Lindsay began to scream. She knew what was happening and she was not happy.

Benn Gilmore was there to greet us and give emotional support. After all, he was an integral part of our family. Since he retired, he recommended Dr. Melissa McBrien to intubate Lindsay for the surgery. Benn commented that she was a dedicated physician and a mom. His opinion meant a great deal to us. Coincidentally, Dr. Greene also recommended Melissa McBrien. She had performed several surgeries on his children as well. We knew we had a winner and someone who would safeguard Lindsay's airway. We met with Dr. McBrien several months prior to the surgery. Lindsay liked her. She even gave her a hug. This was a good sign.

But at this juncture, Lindsay could not be consoled. She knew this was a defining moment and there was no turning back. I could see the look of concern in Benn's eyes as he listened to Lindsay's cries. Benn commented that she had lost weight and looked frail. I knew this saddened him. But we all knew that Lindsay was a fighter and Benn had evidenced this years ago when he saved her life. Lindsay began to calm down when I started to help her undress and get into a hospital gown. She knew this routine and was very cooperative when they inserted the IV. A few nurses recognized Benn and talked with him. When Dr. McBrien entered the pre-op room, Benn took the time to explain Lindsay's anatomy in order to determine the correct type of scope to use during the surgery. Then Dr. Greene came into the room and Jeffrey and I introduced him to Benn. It was quite a friendly atmosphere. We kept talking to Lindsay and she appeared comfortable. I wasn't nervous anymore. I felt a calming presence—I felt that God was with Lindsay and she would be protected. I also knew that God was with Dr. Greene and his entire team. Lindsay would be fine.

We sat in the waiting room and family members filed in during the early morning hours. Their support and love was exactly what was needed. After about a half hour, Dr. Greene came into the waiting area. He said that Lindsay was doing well and then asked about the bone and tissue sample that he was to send to the Netherlands for an associate of Dr. Hennekam's. He inquired if we had a special shipping container that was to be provided by the doctor. I was unaware of the transportation nuances and apparently, both doctors kept missing each other when they tried to discuss this issue. Fortunately, Lindsay's samples could be kept in the anatomical lab until I contacted Dr. Hennekam once again. Lindsay's tissue and bone were to be used in research for the purpose of discovering the cause of advanced bone age and hopefully a remedy to slow down the aging process so individuals can grow to a more natural height. We knew the importance of such research since recently there had been substantial evidence to indicate the first gene that may cause Marshall-Smith Syndrome. It is called NF1X (chromosome 19).

The wait continued for nearly three hours and when Dr. Greene appeared once again he had good news. The hip replacement went well and she now had a plastic and titanium hip. He stated that he secured the hip so that Lindsay would have few restrictions upon her recuperation. He also commented that the incision was glued together for comfort purposes. No pain or irritation would be involved by removal of stitches or staples. Lindsay's airway was fine as well. Dr. Greene had thought of every intricacy so that Lindsay would have an easier time than most recuperating from a total hip replacement.

Lindsay was sent to intensive care after the surgery so that her airway would be closely monitored during the first evening. When several nurses came to alert us that she was in her room, we noted a bit of concern in their voices. Lindsay was somewhat alert and, most likely, not a happy camper nor cooperative. After all, she was probably thinking, "Who are all of these strangers and what is going on?" When we entered her room she had rolled on to her stomach and her legs were bent at the knee, which caused her feet to be in the air. It was quite a sight. She should have been on her back with a wedge between her knees to alleviate pressure on her right leg. She was so happy to see Jeffrey and me, and we helped to calm her down. Lindsay was in a great deal of pain even though she was given medication. Her eyelids began to swell and we were told that it was due to the anesthetic. Lindsay touched my hair and I kissed her. Jeffrey and I were so grateful that the surgery was over and we were now on the road to recovery. Our worst fears had been allayed.

And now I owed God a huge debt. When the surgery was scheduled in July of 2010, I ended my affair with seafood and spareribs to show God that I could follow the laws of *Kashruth*. I still adhere to this routine today. I continually prayed for a successful outcome and I knew that I had to give as well. So I contemplated the various things I could legitimately do and not just say because they sounded good. According to the Torah, *Loshon hara* (gossip) is a terrible offense. It probably rates right up there with murder since gossip can destroy a person's reputation and consequently affect one's life. Well, I never thought of myself as a gossip, at least not a big one. I don't sit around and talk about people, but if the circumstance arises and there's interesting subject matter, then I guess I'm as guilty as the next person. As a result I vowed that I would *work* on this problem and be cognizant of gossip that could ultimately hurt someone. When you stop to think about gossip, you find that it's literally around us all the time. This appeared more difficult than changing some of my food habits. But I embarked on this journey to clean up my act and I am a work in progress. At least I am now aware of this issue the majority of time and I try to remove myself from the situation.

Jeffrey and I stayed with Lindsay the entire time she was in the hospital and rotated to eat and take small breaks. I made Jeffrey go home at night since I knew he would be uncomfortable sleeping in a chair. He's an early riser and was always back before breakfast. Lindsay slept well that first night and there were no issues with her airway. We were now ready to go to the orthopedic floor. Lindsay was pleased to get out of bed and into the wheelchair. She doesn't like to lie around and needs to have action. When we arrived on the floor her bed was not in the room so we walked around and took in the scenery. So many people were recovering from various surgeries. Lindsay enjoyed circling the unit and when her bed arrived she was ready for a break. She'd had some yogurt for breakfast and now she was geared up for something more substantial. We helped her sit in a chair and it was amazing to view the ease with which she simply pushed herself back to get in to a comfortable position. This may seem like an ordinary feat for most individuals, but previously Lindsay would have been in pain trying to do this. Jeffrey and I looked at one another and just smiled. The pain was gone.

On the third morning, when Dr. Greene arrived in Lindsay's room, I asked him if Lindsay could go home. He had previously told us that Lindsay would let us know when she was ready to leave, and after sleeping and eating well, she wasn't about to stay in bed for the day. It was much better to get back into her routine. Dr. Greene gave us his phone number in case we had any issues at home. We left William Beaumont Hospital in the afternoon and Lindsay was a happy camper. She didn't seem to have any discomfort. It appears that the pain she endured for so long was much worse than the hip replacement. She now had to figure out that she could actually put weight on her right leg instead of bending it at the knee and standing on one leg. She needed to remember how to walk.

Physical therapy with Angus began two weeks after Lindsay learned that her right leg could be extended and there would be no pain. We saw this occur while she was sleeping and she definitely seemed more comfortable. Actually, Lindsay began to roll around in bed before finding the right position. She couldn't do this before and was basically in a fetal position, unable to move in fear of pain. Angus stretched Lindsay's muscles and had me walk with her. We paused frequently since she automatically lifted her leg off the ground; it was part of her routine and we needed her to recognize that it was no longer necessary. Angus told me that Lindsay would naturally figure things out in her own time. And he was right! We now can maneuver quite well. Each day she was getting stronger and desired to walk constantly (with assistance). She was even using reciprocal motion, placing one foot and then the other, when going up and down the stairs. Her strides were great and we were totally amazed. She was truly the Bionic Woman.

One month after Lindsay's surgery we had an appointment with Dr. Greene. Lindsay appeared fine in the waiting room until her name was called and we prepared to wheel her in to the examination room. She began to scream and her body became rigid. Taking an x-ray was a chore and then when we entered the room to wait for Dr. Greene, Lindsay proceeded to pull out every bad behavior she knew. She was basically out of control. Maybe she feared another surgery was in the works. Dr. Greene must have heard her since he came in quickly. That was Lindsay's cue to cool it. She calmed down and listened to the conversation.

We viewed her x-rays and saw the prosthetic for the first time. It was quite strange to see this object inserted in Lindsay's femur. Dr. Greene pointed out the two wire clasps, which were added protection for the prosthetic to stay in place. And then Dr. Greene proceeded to tell us about the medical conference he had recently attended. There were approximately 30 orthopedic surgeons and Lindsay's case was presented. The end result of the discussion was this; not one of them would have agreed to perform a total hip replacement. Jeffrey and I were not surprised. Dr. Greene humbly stated that he has no problem helping patients with varying disabilities. He is obviously confident with his craft and, thus, many have benefited from his expertise. In an email from Dr. Zaltz he stated that:

> Perry Greene, by far, has the most experience in Michigan doing joint replacements in small stature patients, and his results are excellent. If you decide to go with the replacement option, he would be my choice over anyone else. I am not recommending him because he is my partner. I always send patients to whom I feel is the most qualified.

Jeffrey and I are certainly thankful for those words of wisdom—even if it took us some time to pull the trigger. Lindsay continues to make progress and she is in such high spirits.. Her laughter is infectious and, as the saying goes, it's apparent that she's one tough customer. On July 1, 2013, there was a repeat performance. This time Lindsay entered the hospital with calm and grace. We had been talking about her surgery for months and she knew it would improve the quality of her life. Lindsay was smiling and laughing. Once again, her other hip was to be replaced by Dr. Greene. This hip was out of the socket and as Dr. Greene stated, "it was flapping in the wind." Basically the same cast of professionals were there again for Lindsay and the results were clear—another successful surgery.

In 1979, when I was expecting Lindsay, I never could have imagined life with a new baby, let alone a child with severe impairments. Every expectant mother is fearful of the new routine and the changes a baby will bring. We all focus on delivering a healthy baby, but somewhere in the recesses of our minds we know exceptions may occur. In retrospect, ever since I heard those three troubling words, "Marshall-Smith Syndrome," fear has been a companion. I've attempted to pack it up and tuck fear away; like placing unwanted items in a storage box. But too often its troublesome head is revealed. We're constantly battling fear of the unknown and it has become a silent occupation. The weight of MSS is daunting, but now I can't imagine life any other way. When Lindsay smiles with delight and her face glows with happiness or when she places her small hand in mine as we walk together, I am truly filled with joy. Lindsay still looks at me with that same expression she had on her face when she was placed in my arms for the first time; and she still speaks to me through her silence and says, "I'm here and I'm not going anywhere." We certainly know there's no crystal ball to foretell what life has in store for us, but we do know that we have been witness to a miracle on several fronts. Jeffrey and I have nothing but profound gratitude for the gifts that Lindsay has brought to our family; we appreciate the best of each day and always have a prayer for tomorrow.

In Memorium

Death is no more than a passing from one room into another. But there's a difference for me, you know. Because in that other room I shall be able to see.
—Helen Keller

Matthew Kayemba Strain, 18 years old
Adam Humphreys, 25 years old

About the Author

Judi Markowitz has been teaching English for 27 years. She instructs 12th graders in the morning at Berkley High School and in the afternoon she teaches a Detroit Film class at CASA (Center for Advanced Studies and the Arts). It's a consortium of six school districts.

She received her Bachelor's Degree in Secondary Education and a Masters Degree in Education Leadership from Wayne State University. Judi is married to Jeffrey Markowitz, her best friend. They live in Huntington Woods, Michigan and have four grown children Lindsay, Chad, Eli, Todd, and daughter-in-law, Chana Tova. They also have three beautiful grand-daughters. *The View From Four Foot Two* is Judi's first published book.

Made in the USA
Charleston, SC
26 February 2014